药学专业
论文
写作

Pharmaceutical
Research
Paper Writing

U0228795

李志裕 主编
吴筱星 副主编

Paper Writing

化学工业出版社
·北京·

内 容 简 介

《药学专业论文写作》结合药学专业论文的各个模块的结构与特点、写作要求与技巧、常见句型与表达等进行分析讲解。全书共分为 10 章内容。第 1 章简要介绍药学文献的基本概念和分类，常见的专业文献检索方法等内容。第 2 章主要探讨科研过程中需要遵循的学术道德和规范，帮助读者树立正确的科学价值观。第 3 章着重介绍标题（Title）的命名原则和写作技巧。第 4 章重点讨论摘要（Abstract）的写作要求和注意事项，并结合实例展示摘要写作的常用表达方式和句型。第 5 章分析了背景介绍（Introduction）部分的写作要素，并进一步分析了文献综述（Review Article）的写作技巧和常见句型。第 6 章着重讨论了实验结果的选取原则和真实准确的呈现方式，阐述了数据处理的基本原则和多样的图表形式。第 7 章分别介绍了讨论（Discussion）与结论（Conclusion）部分的写作要点。第 8 章介绍了论文中实验方法（Method）和补充材料（Supporting Information）部分写作遵循的基本规则。第 9 章着重介绍论文格式规范，并提供论文检查的内容和一般流程。第 10 章介绍了如何进行论文投稿和审稿意见的回复。此外，书后附有常用医药学专业词汇表，辅助药学专业文献阅读与论文写作。

《药学专业论文写作》可作为高等医药类院校药学类专业论文写作课程的指导教材，也可作为药学领域科研工作者撰写论文的参考指南。

图书在版编目（CIP）数据

药学专业论文写作 / 李志裕主编. —北京：化学
工业出版社，2022.3（2022.7 重印）
ISBN 978-7-122-40532-6

Ⅰ. ①药… Ⅱ. ①李… Ⅲ. ①医学–论文–写作
Ⅳ. ①R–05②H152.2

中国版本图书馆 CIP 数据核字（2021）第 273166 号

责任编辑：褚红喜　宋林青	文字编辑：王聪聪　朱　允
责任校对：李雨晴	装帧设计：刘丽华

出版发行：化学工业出版社（北京市东城区青年湖南街 13 号　邮政编码 100011）
印　　装：三河市延风印装有限公司
710mm×1000mm　1/16　印张 11½　字数 202 千字　2022 年 7 月北京第 1 版第 2 次印刷

购书咨询：010-64518888　　　　　　　　售后服务：010-64518899
网　　址：http://www.cip.com.cn

凡购买本书，如有缺损质量问题，本社销售中心负责调换。

定　　价：39.80 元

《药学专业论文写作》
编写人员

主　编　李志裕

副 主 编　吴筱星

编写人员（按姓氏笔画排列）

刘东飞　孙昊鹏　孙晓莲

李志裕　肖易倍　吴春勇

吴筱星　郑秋凌　戴　丽

前言

　　对于药学专业的学生和研究者来说，专业文献的研读和写作是必不可少的，这既是获取专业药学知识、跟踪药学研究前沿的重要渠道，也是进行科研交流的主要方式之一。现今社会，每天都有大量的新研究发现被报道，药学领域亦然。电子信息化和网络的普及，为这些知识成果的存储和传播提供了极为便捷的途径。要想从这些海量的信息中获取相关专业知识，提高文献检索的效率和质量，则需要药学工作者掌握专门的工具及方法。同样，对获取的文献进行研读，也需要具备相关的药学知识和研读的方法技巧。特别是，如果药学研究者需要流畅地撰写专业论文，除了遵循一定的语言规范外，还需掌握论文各个板块的写作要点和方法技巧。

　　本书共分为10章，对药学专业论文的各个模块进行剖析讲解，结合各自模块的特点介绍其写作要求和常用技巧，并在书后附有药学专业词汇表。第1章为课程概述，简要地介绍药学文献的基本概念和分类，常见的专业文献获取方法，以及期刊的通用评价方式。第2章主要探讨科研过程中需要遵循的学术道德和规范，包括对实验数据的正确处理、科研结果的规范发表、他人成果的合理引用等，并结合具体的实例指出违反学术诚信的表现形式和严重后果，帮助树立正确的科学价值观。第3章着重介绍标题（Title）部分的命名原则和写作技巧，学术论文的标题短小精悍，必须做到字字珠玑，以至字体和大小写都需格外注意。此外，还列举了常见的标题范式和该部分写作需要规避的禁忌。第4章重点讨论摘要（Abstract）的写作要求和注意事项，指明摘要的作用和内容，并结合实例展示摘要写作的常用表达方式和句型。第5章为背景介绍（Introduction）部分的写作，该部分内容包括研究主题、学术重要性、文献调研、知识缺口、研究问题、研究成果及贡献六要素，并进一步分析了文献调研的写作技巧和常见句型。第6章着重讨论实验结果（Results）和数据处理，讨论了实验结果的选取原则和真实准确的呈现方式，阐述了数据处理的基本原则和多样的图表形式。第7章分别介绍了讨论（Discussion）与结论（Conclusion）部分的写作要点，讨论部分的写作应与已有结果做充分的比较，以体现作者自身研究的重要性和差异性；结论部分的写作需特别注意其与摘要的异同点。第8章为实验方法（Method）和补充材料（Supporting Information），该部分写作一般遵循"基本，简洁，不做结论"的规则。第9章着重介绍论文格式规范和手稿材料检查，是论文投稿前的必需步骤，列举了英语写作中的常见句式和容易忽略的错误，提供论文检查的内容和一般流程。第10章为论文投稿和审稿意见回复，包括投稿前的准备工作，投稿信（Cover Letter）的写作要点，以及如何有理有据有节地回复审稿人意见。

本书从药学专业文献的写作着手，提供大量的药学专业论文实例，并结合文献的检索和研读，给广大药学工作者提供相关的药学文献知识和写作方法，以达到通过专业文献丰富自身知识架构和促进科研交流的目的。

本书是基于中国药科大学药学院药物化学、药剂学、药理学、药物分析学四个药学专业方向的"药学专业文献与论文写作"课程的讲义上成稿的，在编写过程中得到诸多同事的帮助和支持，同时，在本书编写过程中引用了相关国内外文献资料，在此一并向他们表示衷心的感谢。限于编者的水平，书中不妥之处在所难免，恳请读者批评指正。

编　者

2021年5月于南京

目录

第 1 章

课程概述

第 2 章

科研诚信和道德规范

第 3 章

标题

第 4 章

摘要

第 5 章

背景介绍

第 6 章

实验结果与数据处理

第 7 章

讨论与结论

第 8 章

实验方法与补充材料

第 9 章

论文格式规范及检查

第 10 章

论文投稿及审稿意见回复

第 1 章 ●○

课程概述

本章将主要介绍药学专业文献的概念和类型、代表性的药学专业期刊、常用的文献检索方式和工具。其次，讨论如何合理地运用影响因子、H指数（H-index）等指标，对专业期刊及研究者做出较为公正的评价。最后补充一些药学专业论文写作前的基本知识和准备工作，以达到对专业文献研读与写作的初步了解。

1.1 药学专业文献的类型

根据国家标准局（NBS）的界定，**文献**就是指记录有知识的一切载体，它包括三要素：**载体**（媒介）、**知识**（信息）、**表达方式**（文字、图像、声音和符号等）。其中，知识是文献的实质内容，载体是文献的外在形式，而表达方式是知识与载体的相互联系。文献的种类有多种多样，在药学专业领域主要有专业图书、专业期刊、专利文献、科技报告、会议文献、学位论文等。

（1）专业图书

专业图书是一类总结性的、经过重新组织的二次和三次文献。它包括教科书、专著、评论书、方法书、科学读物以及参考工具书，而参考工具书又包括词典、手册、百科全书等。

例如：

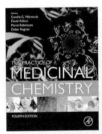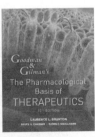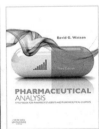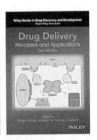

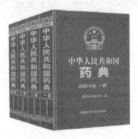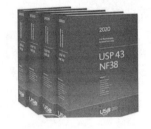

扫码看高清彩图

国家药典是药品的国家标准，我国除《中华人民共和国药典》外，还有中华人民共和国国家卫生健康委员会药品标准，各省自治区、直辖市药品标准，规定了药品的质量标准和检验方法。2002年国家开始清理并取消地方标准。现行《中华人民共和国药典》（简称《中国药典》）分为四部出版：一部收载药材和饮片、植物油脂和提取物、成方制剂和单味制剂等；二部收载化学药品、抗生素、生化药品以及放射性药品等；三部收载生物制品；四部收载通则，包括制剂通则、检验方法、指导原则、标准物质和试液试药相关通则、药用辅料等。

（2）专业期刊

期刊又称杂志（Journal，Magazine），以发表科研方面的论文为主，具有较强的学术性，是科技文献的主体。一般是指具有固定题名、定期或不定期出版的连续出版物，不预定何时终止，无限期地发行，卷、期号、出版时间相对稳定。专业期刊具有以下特点：

① 期刊所载文章一般都是由不同著者所写，独立成篇，互不相关。

② 周期相对固定。一般有周刊、旬刊、半月刊、月刊、双月刊、季刊和年刊等，有时还出版临时特刊、专刊或附录。例如，药物化学的权威期刊 *Journal of Medicinal Chemistry*，隶属于美国化学会（American Chemical Society，ACS），连续定期出版，为半月刊。

③ 科技期刊的名称也不完全统一，一般以学科名称加"杂志""学报""通报"等命名，如《药学学报》《化学学报》《中华医学杂志》等；英文名称也较复杂，有的以学科英文名称冠以如 *"Journal of""Acta of" "Bulletin of""Archives of"* 等期刊或杂志字样，也有不加期刊或杂志等字样的，直接以学科名称命名，如 *Cell*、*Nature*、*Science* 等。

④ 出版周期短、速度快、刊载论文多、内容新颖，能比较及时地反映世界科技发展的水平和动向。目前，在科学技术界已形成了通过科技期刊发表科研成就的传统，许多新的成果、新的观点、新的方法往往首先在期刊上刊登，已是科学交流的主要工具。

根据科技期刊的特点和调研工作的内容，所发表的论文通常可以分为以下几类，这些也是本书主要探讨写作的论文题材。

① Original research articles/Full paper：原创科研，详细工作。

② Short/Rapid/Brief Communication：原创科研，短小精悍且创新性强。

③ Letters：更短的原创科研。

④ Review（Mini Review，Perspcctive）：对现有论文的总结综述。

⑤ Comments/Editorial Materials：对现有某一工作的评论。

（3）专利文献

专利文献主要指专利说明书，是指专利申请人向政府登记时递交的能说明创造发明内容的书面文件。一般来说，专利申请要经过新颖性、创造性、实用性审查，对科技人员而言，专利文献是具体而有启发性的重要参考文献。新的专利文献可以反映当时科技发展的最新水平，并可以通过它预测出新技术发展的动向。

药物专利的授予：一种是新化合物的发现和合成方法，以及针对某类靶点/疾病的应用，全球多数国家都会授予专利保护，可以在专利文献中查阅获取原文；另一种是药用物质的制剂工艺等，有的国家授予专利保护，有的国家不授予专利保护，不受专利保护的国家的制剂工艺情报，就无法在专利文献中查找。

（4）科技报告

科技报告（特指政府出版的科技报告）也是连续出版物，但每期只收载一篇报告，是政府出版物的一种。科技报告又分专题报告、专人报告及年度科技报告等，在检索工具的文摘中，常有"Report"标志。其目的是向上级主管部门汇报某一领域的发展动态，并给予必要的建议。每份单独成册，有专门的编号，其特点有：

① 内容具体；

② 有科研项目的研究方案、实验记录、实验数据、图表等；

③ 报道比期刊早；

④ 保密或控制发行。

（5）会议文献

会议文献是指国际学术会议和各国国内重要学术会议上发表的论文和报告。一般都要经过学术机构严格的挑选，代表某学科领域的最新成就，反映该学科领域的最新水平和发展趋势。所以会议文献是了解国际及各国的科技水平、动态及发展趋势的重要情报文献。但会议文献与期刊及其他类型的文献有重复交叉。例如：催化会议、有机化学会议、美国化学会年会（American Chemical Society Annual Meeting）、NPRA（National Petrochemical &

Refiners Association）等会议文献资料。

（6）学位论文

学位论文是为了取得博士（Doctor）、硕士（Master）、学士（Bachelor）等学位进行答辩时撰写的科学论文。常有"Diss."（Dissertation 的缩写）标志，而且有学位论文编号，如 Order NO. DA 8328940 From Diss. Abstr. Int. B 1984，44（8）：2428.

1.2　药学专业期刊介绍

1.2.1　药学专业的综述性期刊

药学专业的综述性期刊主要有如下：

① 自然出版集团（Nature Publishing Groups，NPG）：出版多个药学和医学专业领域的综述类期刊。

Nature Reviews（《自然评论》）系列期刊主要有：

Nature Reviews Cancer，*Nature Reviewrs Cardiology*，*Nature Reviews Chemistry*，*Nature Reviews Clinical Oncology*，*Nature Reviews Disease Primers*，*Nature Reviews Drug Discovery*，*Nature Reviews Endocrinology*，*Nature Reviews Gastroenterology & Hepatology*，*Nature Reviews Genetics*，*Nature Reviews Immunology*，*Nature Reviews Materials*，*Nature Reviews Microbiology*，*Nature Reviews Molecular Cell Biology*，*Nature Reviews Nephrology*，*Nature Reviews Neurology*，*Nature Reviews Neuroscience*，*Nature Reviews Rheumatology*，*Nature Reviews Urology*。

② *Chemical Reviews*：由美国化学会（ACS）出版的化学综述类期刊。

③ *Chemical Society Reviews*：由英国皇家化学会（RSC）出版的化学综述类期刊。

④ *Trends in Pharmacological Sciences*：由荷兰爱思唯尔（Elsevier）旗下的细胞出版社（Cell Press）出版的药学综述类期刊。

⑤ *Medicinal Research Reviews*：由美国威利（Wiley）出版社出版的药学综述类期刊。

⑥ *Drug Discovery Today*：由荷兰爱思唯尔（Elsevier）出版的药学综述类期刊。

⑦ *Advanced Drug Delivery Reviews*：由荷兰爱思唯尔（Elsevier）出版的药剂学综述类期刊。

⑧ *Annual Review of Pharmacology and Toxicology*：由美国 Annual Reviews 出版的药理学和毒理学综述类期刊。

⑨ *Pharmacological Reviews*：由美国药理学和实验治疗学会（American Society for Pharmacology and Experimental Therapeutics）出版的药理学及相关的综述类期刊。

1.2.2 药学专业的研究性论文期刊（综合类）

药学专业的研究性论文期刊（综合类）主要有如下：

① *Cell*

② *Nature*

③ *Science*

④ *Journal of American Chemical Society*

⑤ *Angewandte Chemie International Edition*

⑥ *Nature Communications*

⑦ *Nature Metabolism*

⑧ *Nature Medicine*

⑨ *Nature Chemical Biology*

⑩ *Acta Pharmaceutica Sinica B*

其中，*Cell*、*Nature*、*Science*、*Journal of American Chemical Society*、*Angewandte Chemie International Edition* 和 *Acta Pharmaceutica Sinica B* 的封面风格如下所示。

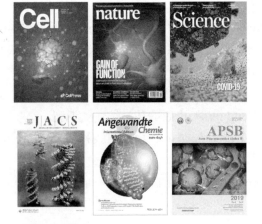

扫码看高清彩图

1.2.3　药学专业的研究性论文期刊（以药学专业分类）

根据药学专业分类，药学专业的研究性论文期刊主要可分为药物化学主流期刊、药物分析主流期刊、药理学主流期刊、药剂学主流期刊。

（1）药物化学主流期刊

① *Journal of Medicinal Chemistry*

② *European Journal of Medicinal Chemistry*

③ *ACS Medicinal Chemistry Letters*

④ *Bioorganic & Medicinal Chemistry*

⑤ *Bioorganic & Medicinal Chemistry Letters*

⑥ *ChemMedChem*

⑦ *Future Medicinal Chemistry*

⑧ *Current Medicinal Chemistry*

上述 8 种药物化学主流期刊的封面如下所示。

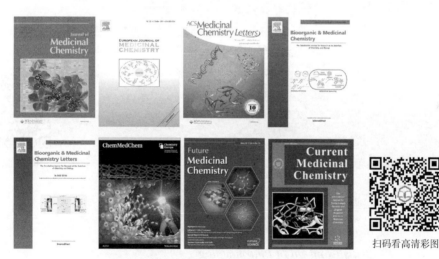

扫码看高清彩图

（2）药物分析主流期刊

① *Analytical Chemistry*

② *Analytical Methods*

③ *Analytica Chimica Acta*

④ *Journal of Mass Spectrometry*

⑤ *Journal of Chromatography A*

⑥ *Journal of Proteome Research*

⑦ *Journal of Pharmaceutical and Biomedical Analysis*

⑧ *Journal of Chromatography B*

上述部分药物分析主流期刊的封面如下所示。

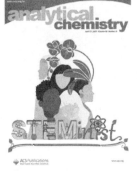
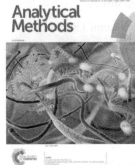
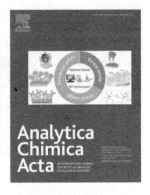
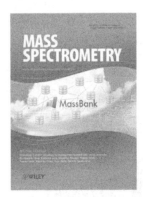
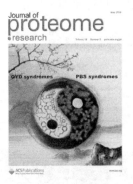
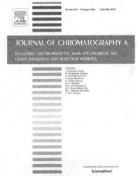

扫码看高清彩图

（3）药理学主流期刊

① *Biochemical Pharmacology*

② *British Journal of Pharmacology*

③ *Frontiers in Pharmacology*

④ *Molecular Pharmaceutics*

⑤ *Neuro pharmacology*

⑥ *Pharmacological Research*

上述 6 种药理学主流期刊的封面如下所示。

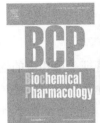
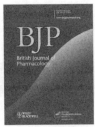

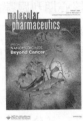
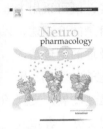
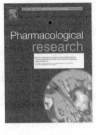

扫码看高清彩图

（4）药剂学主流期刊

① *Journal of Controlled Release*

② *Journal of Pharmaceutical Sciences*

③ *Pharmaceutical Research*

④ *Molecular Pharmaceutics*

⑤ *European Journal of Pharmaceutical Sciences*

⑥ *Asian Journal of Pharmaceutical Sciences*

⑦ *The Journal of Physical Chemistry B*

上述 7 种药剂学主流期刊的封面如下所示。

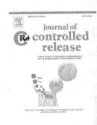
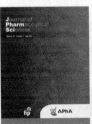
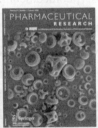
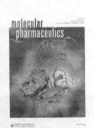
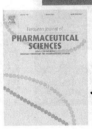
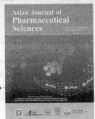
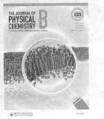

扫码看高清彩图

1.3　药学文献检索

　　文献检索一般根据文献的外部特征和内容特征采用相应的途径，其中根据文献的外部特征可采取文献名途径、作者途径、序号途径等，根据文献的内容特征可采取主题途径、关键词途径、结构途径、学科分类途径等。文献检索的方法也形式多样，既可采用专业核心期刊跟踪的**直检法**，也可采用论文参考文献和引用目录的**追溯法**，以及根据课题研究年份由远及近的**顺查法**和研究年份由近及远的**倒查法**，力求在最短的时间、以最有效的方式满足知识积累和课题研究的文献需求。

　　随着互联网和科学研究的迅速发展，文献的更新频繁，且规模空前。同时，学科之间相互交融，使得文献内容重复交叉，又分布离散。传统依赖于目录、题录、文摘和主题词检索已不能适应新形势的要求。高效查找到可靠文献成为药学研究者的基本技能。

1.3.1　美国国家生物技术信息中心（https://www.ncbi.nlm.nih.gov）

　　美国国家生物技术信息中心（National Center for Biotechnology Information，NCBI）是美国国家医学图书馆（NLM）的下属机构（该图书馆是美国国立卫生研究所的一部分），是世界上重要的生物信息数据库之一，包括基因、基因组、蛋白质信息，以及临床及小分子化合物相关信息。通过其官方网站网址可一站式快捷检索。

　　（1）PubMed（https://pubmed.ncbi.nlm.nih.gov/）

　　PubMed 是由 NCBI 提供的免费文摘型数据库，是以生物医药信息为核心的检索系统。PubMed 数据库包含超过 3200 万份生物医学文献的引文和摘要，并提供期刊原文链接。

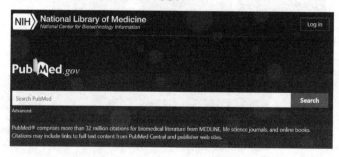

扫码看高清彩图

（2）PubChem（https://pubchem.ncbi.nlm.nih.gov/）

PubChem 是 NCBI 于 2004 年开发的以小分子为主的生物活性免费数据库，数据库包括 3 个子数据库：① PubChem BioAssay，提供生物活性测定实验方法等相关数据；② PubChem Compound，以化合物化学结构为标识的化合物信息数据库；③ PubChem Substance，提供以物质名称为标识的化合物数据库。PubChem 可以按化合物名称、分子式、结构和其他标识符检索化学物质的化学和物理性质、生物活性、安全性和毒性信息，以及相关专利、文献引用等。目前可供检索的具有确定化学结构的化合物有 1.1 亿种，化学实体信息 2.7 亿种，生物活性数据 2.9 亿种，相关文献 3300 万篇，专利 3000 万篇，并在不断持续增加。

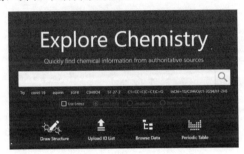

扫码看高清彩图

1.3.2　Web of Science（http://apps.webofknowledge.com）

Web of Science 是 Clarivate Analytics（科睿唯安，原汤森路透知识产权与科技）开发的以自然科学为主的收费文献检索数据库，数据来源于期刊、图书、专利、会议录、网络资源（包括免费开放资源）等。它是最早以引文数据为指标来评价论文、期刊、文献著者、科研机构的数据库，因此通过该数据库可以查找高水平的论文、著者及机构。

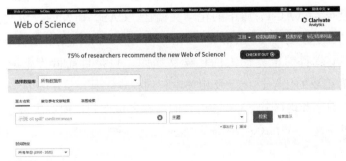

扫码看高清彩图

1.3.3 药物早期研发情报数据库（CDDI）(https://www.cortellis.com/drug discovery/)

它是由科睿唯安开发的收费数据库，收录自 1988 以来的药物早期研发必需的生物学、化学和药理学信息，通过整合 60 万有生物活性的化学分子和生物分子，涉及疾病领域综述、实验药理学、动物模型、药代动力学/代谢相关实验数据、SAR 构效关系、靶点和相关通路信息、临床试验信息等。以集成报告、动画解说、靶标通路图等各种易于接受的形式进行信息传递，为新药研发人员提供独特的知识解决方案，以支持药物研发活动。下图为 CDDI 检索冠状病毒（coronavirus）所给出的全景图。

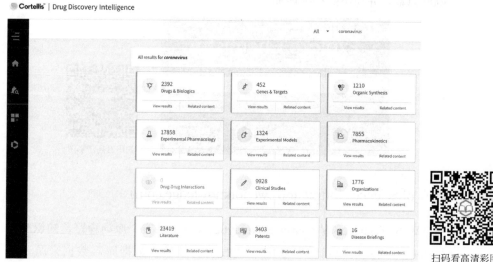

扫码看高清彩图

1.3.4 SciFinder (https://scifinder.cas.org)

SciFinder（需要付费账号登录，使用前请先咨询所在学校或单位）是由美国化学会（ACS）旗下的化学文摘社（CAS）研发的收费文摘型数据库，它的前身是 CAS 出版的《化学文摘》（*Chemical Abstract*，简称 CA）。CA 是目前世界最大的化学文摘库，也是目前世界上应用最为广泛、最为重要的化学、化工及相关学科的检索工具。SciFinder 综合了全球 200 多个国家和地区的 60 多种语言的 1 万多份期刊，内容丰富全面。使用者能通过主题、分子式、结构式和反应式等多种方式进行检索，并提供全文链接。

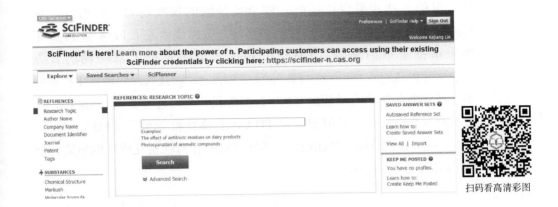

扫码看高清彩图

1.3.5 Reaxys （https://www.reaxys.com）

Reaxys 数据库是由爱思唯尔（Elsevier）公司研发的收费数据库，是目前全球最大、数据架构最完整的药物化学数据库。Reaxys 将贝尔斯坦（Beilstein）、专利化学数据库（Patent）和盖墨林（Gmelin）的内容整合为统一的资源，包含了 5400 多万个反应、1.4 亿种物质、400 多万条生物活性数据，可提供靶点、活性等级、临床研发状态、机制、药物代谢及结构等多种方式进行检索。

扫码看高清彩图

1.3.6 药物研发与监管科学数据库 （https://www.pharmapendium.com/home）

药物研发与监管科学数据库（PharmaPendium）是由爱思唯尔（Elsevier）公司研发针对上市药物的收费数据库，提供上市药物的临床前与临床、药效、药物安全及药代动力学、药物代谢与转运酶、药物不良反应报告等数据的一站式平台；同时还收录此领域的权威期刊书籍内容，如 Meyler 副反应大全和 Mosby 用药参考等。数据库涵盖了 FDA 从 1938 年以来审批上市的药物，EMA 从 1995 年以来审批上市药物的官方 Approval Package、Advisory Committee Report，以及从这些报告中提取的关于药物的药代动力学数据（PK）、新陈代谢与转运体数据（MET）、药效数据（Efficacy），同时整合了 FDA 不良事件报告系统（FDA Adverse Effect Report System，FAERS），并且可以进行药物相互作用的风险预测（DDI Risk Calculator）。

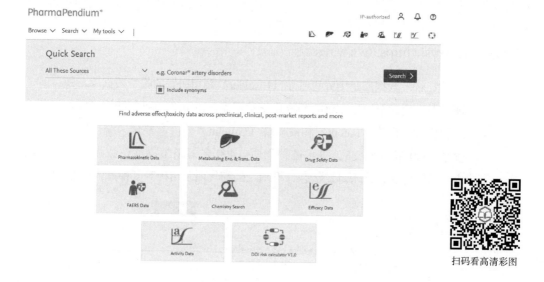

扫码看高清彩图

1.3.7 药物临床研发情报数据库（Pharm Intelligence）（https://citeline.informa.com/）

药物临床研发情报数据库（Pharm Intelligence）是 Informa 公司提供的药物全周期数据库，包含三个模块：Pharmaprojects、Sitetrove、Trialtrove。可以全面了解到各种原研药从临床前到上市的全部历史研发记录、各国许可信息、各国上市信息、不同适应证的研发阶段等。

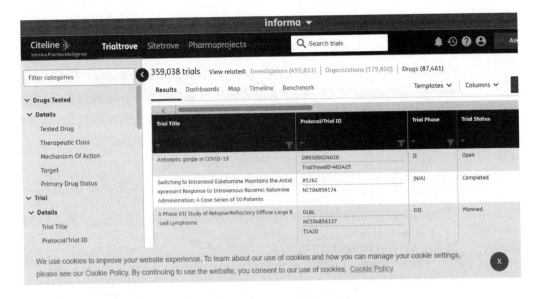

1.3.8　ScienceDirect（https://www.sciencedirect.com）

ScienceDirect 是爱思唯尔的收费全文数据库，是目前全世界最大的科学、科技特别是医学全文与书目电子资源数据库，超过全球核心期刊品种的 25%，包含 3800 多种同行评审期刊与 37000 多本电子书，共有 1400 余万篇文献。

1.3.9　EBSCOhost（http://search.ebscohost.com/）

EBSCOhost 是由著名文献出版机构 EBSCO 提供，包括自然科学、社会科学、人文和艺术科学等各类学科领域的期刊、图书等收费全文数据库。其中收录的期刊有一半以上是 SCI、SSCI 的来源期刊，是世界上收录学科比较齐全的全文期刊联机数据库。

1.3.10　SpringerLink（https://link.springer.com/）

施普林格（Springer）是世界著名的科技期刊、图书出版公司。SpringerLink 按学科分为 13 个子数据库，可提供电子图书、期刊的全文检索。其旗下的自然出版集团拥有以 *Nature* 为代表的一系列与药物研发相关的高水平期刊。

1.3.11　OVID（http://ovidsp.ovid.com）

OVID 是 OVID Technologies 提供的以医学为主导的收费全文数据库。

该数据库主要包括世界第二大医学出版社 Lippincott Williams & Wilkins（LWW）及英国医学学会系列电子全文数据库（BMA Journals Fulltext）、牛津大学出版社医学电子全文数据库（OUP Journals Fulltext）。其中 Drug Information Fulltext 数据库包含 AHFS 药物信息数据库，广泛收录了药物相互作用、用法和毒性的全面分析、药物剂量和管理办法的详细信息、药物化学性和稳定性的调查报告以及药理学和药物代谢动力学相关数据。

1.3.12　美国化学会期刊数据库（https://pubs.acs.org/）

美国化学会期刊数据库是 ACS（American Chemical Society）旗下的期刊全文收费数据库。ACS 出版的化学及药学相关学科期刊很多是各学科领域里高水平的代表。现按 6 大学科分类，出版近百种期刊和图书，最早可以追溯到 1879 年。

1.3.13　中国知网（https://www.cnki.net/）

中国知网由清华大学、清华同方发起，始建于 1999 年 6 月。数据库内容覆盖自然科学、工程技术、农业、哲学、医学、人文社会科学等各个领域，囊括了基础研究、工程技术、行业指导、党政工作、文化生活、科学普及等各层次的期刊。

1.3.14　X-MOL（https://www.x-mol.com）

X-MOL 是一款传播和检索科学知识的平台，拥有学术期刊、行业信息、海外导师、网站导航等多种功能内容，可以帮助研究者更好地进行信息检索和学习。

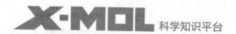

英文期刊搜索，请输入：英文关键词、作者名、DOI或期刊名＋年＋卷＋页码　　文献搜索　　高级检索

1.3.15　欧洲专利局专利文献数据库（https://worldwide.espacenet.com）

欧洲专利局专利文献数据库是由欧洲专利局免费提供的在线专利数据

库，包含多种专利检索、全文下载、法律状态查询以及审查过程、文档查询等信息服务。

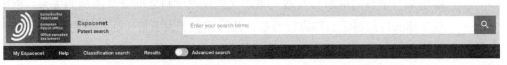

Espacenet: free access to over 120 million patent documents

值得一提的是，为了方便识别和检索文献，当前每篇药学科技论文都会有一个数字对象标识符（Digital Object Identifier，DOI），相当于科技论文的身份证，具有唯一性。通过 DOI 可以方便、可靠地链接到论文全文，从而确保了网络环境下对特定数字化论文的准确提取，有效地避免重复或遗漏。此外，论文的 DOI 标识符一经产生就永久不变，不随其所标识的数字化对象的版权所有者或存储地址等属性的变更而改变。一个 DOI 通常包括两个部分：前缀和后缀，中间用"/"分割。前缀由两部分组成，起始是一个"10."的目录代码，紧接着是组织或单位向 IDF 申请的登记机构代码。后缀是一个在特定前缀下唯一的后缀，由登记机构分配并确保其唯一性。后缀可以是任何字母数字码，其编码方案完全由登记机构自己来规定。后缀可以是一个机器码，或者是一个已有的规范码，如 ISBN 号或 ISSN号。药学专业论文的 DOI 号一般出现在论文主页或文中。

例：图中所示论文的 DOI 号出现在标题页的右上角。

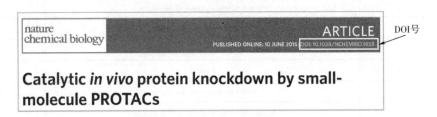

1.4 期刊及研究者的评价方式

1.4.1 科学引文索引和影响因子

科学引文索引（Science Citation Index，SCI）是由美国科学信息研究所

（ISI）于 1961 年创办出版的引文数据库，是目前国际上被公认的最具权威性的科技文献检索数据库。引文索引系统打破了传统的学科分类界限，既能揭示某一学科的继承与发展关系，又能反映学科之间交叉渗透的关系。SCI 对全球的自然科学刊物进行考察，凡影响因子大于某一临界值的刊物，则可以进入 SCI 系统。进入 SCI 系统的刊物分为两类：内圈和外圈。前者的影响因子高于后者，前者称为 SCI 刊物，后者称为 SCIsearch 刊物。

影响因子（Impact Factor，IF）是美国科学信息研究所的《期刊引证报告》（Journal Citation Reports，JCR）中的一项数据，是国际上通行的评价期刊学术水平和论文质量的重要指标。影响因子以年度为单位进行计算，即某期刊前两年发表的论文在该报告年份（JCR year）中被引用总次数除以该期刊在这两年内发表的论文总数。许多著名学术期刊会在其网站上注明期刊的影响因子，以表明在对应学科的影响力。如果一位研究者能经常在高影响因子的期刊上发表论文，则能部分反映该研究者的科研水平，但不可以此为单一标准。SCI 的影响因子一般于每年的 6 月份公布，由 Thomson Reuters 统计发布，此为最准确的官方版本，其他网站均以此为版本，只作为参考意义，并非百分之百准确。表 1-1 是 2020 年影响因子排名前二十的期刊。

※ 表 1-1　2020 年影响因子排名前二十期刊

排名	期刊名称	IF
1	*CA：A Cancer Journal for Clinicians*	292.3
2	*New England Journal of Medicine*	74.7
3	*Nature Reviews Materials*	71.2
4	*Nature Reviews Drug Discovery*	64.8
5	*Lancet*	60.4
6	*WHO Technical Report Series*	59.0
7	*Nature Reviews Molecular Cell Biology*	55.5
8	*Nature Reviews Clinical Oncology*	53.3
9	*Nature Reviews Cancer*	53.0
10	*Chemical Reviews*	52.8
11	*Nature Energy*	46.5
12	*JAMA–Journal of The American Medical Association*	45.5
13	*Reviews of Modern Physics*	45.0
14	*Chemical Society Reviews*	42.9

排名	期刊名称	IF
15	*Nature*	42.8
16	*Science*	41.9
17	*Nature Reviews Disease Primers*	40.7
18	*World Psychiatry*	40.6
19	*Nature Reviews Immunology*	40.4
20	*Nature Materials*	38.7

期刊的影响因子每年都会有变化，而是否被 SCI 收录也存在着动态调整，一些期刊由于以下原因而被剔除在 SCI 之外：

① 论文质量普遍差，影响因子常年极低；

② 审稿机制存在严重缺陷，导致大量审稿造假；

③ 收取高额版面费，文章接受率高，发文量大幅增长，有掠夺性期刊嫌疑；

④ 自引率太高，有刷高影响因子的嫌疑。

1.4.2 中科院期刊分区

中科院 JCR 期刊分区是中国科学院文献情报中心科学前沿分析中心每年发布一次的期刊分区，旨在纠正当时国内科研界对不同学科期刊影响因子数值差异的误解，是通过 JCR 中 SCI 期刊在学科内依据 3 年平均影响因子划分分区。中科院期刊分区包括大类分区和小类分区。大类学科是在充分考虑国内科研和教育体系的特点所设置的，分别为数学、物理、化学、地学、地学天文、生物学、农林科学、医学、工程技术、环境科学与生态学、管理科学、社会科学。大类分区包括 Top 期刊；而小类分区是将期刊按照 JCR 已有学科分类体系所做的分区。表 1-2 是药学类相关 SCI 期刊 2017—2019 三年间的影响因子。

※ 表 1-2 药学类相关 SCI 期刊 2017—2019 三年间的影响因子

期刊名称	中科院分区	2017 IF	2018 IF	2019 IF
Journal of The American Chemical Society	化学 1 区	14.4	14.7	14.6
Angewandte Chemie International Edition	化学 1 区	12.1	12.3	13.0
Chemical Communications	化学 1 区	6.3	6.2	6.0

期刊名称	中科院分区	2017 IF	2018 IF	2019 IF
British Journal of Pharmacology	药学 1 区	6.8	6.9	7.7
Alimentary Pharmacology & Therapeutics	药学 1 区	7.4	7.7	7.5
Acta Pharmaceutica Sinica B	药学 1 区	6.0	5.8	7.1
Neuropsychopharmacology	药学 1 区	6.5	7.2	6.8
Clinical Pharmacology & Therapeutics	药学 1 区	6.5	6.4	6.6
Journal of Medicinal Chemistry	药物化学 1 区	6.3	6.0	6.2
European Journal of Medicinal Chemistry	药物化学 1 区	4.8	4.8	5.6
Organic Letters	有机化学 1 区	6.5	6.6	6.1
Organic Chemistry Frontiers	有机化学 1 区	5.5	5.1	5.2
Acta Pharmacologica Sinica	药学 2 区	3.6	4.0	5.1
Biochemical Pharmacology	药学 2 区	4.2	4.8	5.0
Current Opinion in Pharmacology	药学 2 区	6.3	5.2	4.8
CNS Drugs	药学 2 区	4.2	4.2	4.8
Journal of Food and Drug Analysis	药学 2 区	2.9	4.2	4.7
Current Neuropharmacology	药学 2 区	4.1	4.6	4.7
Neuropharmacology	药学 2 区	4.2	4.4	4.4
Frontiers in Pharmacology	药学 2 区	3.8	3.8	4.2
Vascular Pharmacology	药学 2 区	3.6	3.3	4.1
Journal of Neuroimmune Pharmacology	药学 2 区	3.7	3.9	4.1
Asian Journal of Pharmacology Sciences	药学 2 区	4.6	4.0	4.0
British Journal of Clinical Pharmacology	药学 2 区	3.8	3.9	3.7
Chemico-Biological Interactions	药学 2 区	3.3	3.4	3.7
Molecular Pharmacology	药学 2 区	4.0	3.9	3.7
European Journal of Pharmaceutical Sciences	药学 2 区	3.5	3.5	3.6
Journal of Pharmacology and Experimental Therapeutics	药学 2 区	3.7	3.6	3.6
Toxicology and Applied Pharmacology	药学 2 区	3.7	3.6	3.3
Pharmaceutical Research	药学 2 区	3.3	3.9	3.2
Journal of Enzyme Inhibition and Medicinal Chemistry	药物化学 2 区	3.6	4.0	4.7
ACS Medicinal Chemistry Letters	药物化学 2 区	3.8	3.7	4.0
Journal of Natural Products	药物化学 2 区	3.9	4.3	3.8
Future Medicinal Chemistry	药物化学 2 区	4.0	3.6	3.6
Bioorganic Chemistry	化学 2 区	3.9	3.9	4.8
Chinese Chemical Letters	化学 2 区	2.6	3.8	4.6

1.4.3 H指数

H指数（H-index）又称为H因子（H-factor），是一种评价科研人员学术成就的方法。H代表"高引用次数"（high citations），一名科研人员的H指数是指他至多有H篇论文分别被引用了至少H次。H指数能够比较准确地反映一个人的学术成就。一个人的H指数越高，则表明他的论文影响力越大。

1.5 药学专业论文的写作准备

撰写一篇药学专业论文之前，研究者应该确保研究的内容和结果是具有原创性的（综述论文除外），对本领域具有一定程度的贡献。同时，对论文的写作应该有一个初步的认识，需要掌握一些基本的法则。

（1）留出充足的时间进行构思和书写手稿

手稿撰写所花费的时间应该是跟该科学研究所花费的精力呈正相关的。如果时间过于仓促，则可能会导致对该领域的背景调查不够充分，写作思路出现偏差，论文中出现多处低级错漏，从而使原本取得的优秀科研成果被低估而拒稿。

（2）选择内容合适的期刊，并尽量选择影响因子较高的或者是专业内的旗舰期刊

根据自身的研究内容和实验结果，选择符合要求的期刊。如前所述，影响因子是衡量一份期刊声望的重要标准，影响因子越高其读者就越多；相应的，其他研究者引用论文的可能性就越大，则自身的研究更容易得到同行的关注。当然，在高影响因子期刊上发表论文的难度也会增大，所以也要切忌好高骛远。

（3）仔细阅读所选期刊的作者指南和下载论文的写作模板

每个期刊都有各自的要求和风格特点。作者在写作之前应先仔细阅读作者指南，深入理解该期刊对论文架构、格式规范、投稿材料、图表内容等方面做出的指导性规定，并严格按照所选期刊的作者指南进行论文撰写

和材料准备。在手稿撰写时，尽量采用期刊推荐的模板，包括对论文的字数限制、字体大小、标题格式、图表形式、参考文献引用等。

（4）设定论文各部分的写作顺序，并按照由粗略到精细的过程打磨

对于初次写作的作者来说，可以借鉴以下常见的写作顺序：摘要、方法、实验结果、讨论、背景介绍、结论。总体来说，方法和实验结果部分的写作难度较低，而背景介绍和讨论是难度较大的写作部分。

（5）选择多篇本领域的优秀论文进行精读

精读优秀论文，记下有用的短语和句型，并选择其中一篇论文作为模板，用于前期套用，在后续的修改稿中逐渐脱离其窠臼。

（6）与本领域的研究者进行交流

把自己的研究结果和重要发现整理出来，与不同层次的研究者进行交流。交流对象既可以是刚踏上科研之路的研究生，也可以是资深的专家教授，听取他们对该研究的意见和建议，以及手稿写作的思路。

（7）时刻牢记审稿人

手稿撰写过程中应该时刻牢记审稿人，要从他们的角度考虑：①研究内容是否吻合期刊的一贯风格？②该研究发现是否足够重要？③实验结果和结论是否完整准确？并在必要的时候及时补充关键的实验数据。

课后练习与讨论

1. 请指出研究性期刊和综述类期刊的区别，并根据药学专业分类分别列举 3 种期刊。
2. 药物化学、药物分析、药理学以及药剂学专业的主流期刊分别有哪些？
3. 一篇科技论文的唯一编号被称作什么？它有什么特点和作用？
4. 期刊的影响因子取决于哪些因素？如何正确地对待影响因子？
5. 如何进行有效的文献检索？试用实例加以演示和说明。

第 2 章 ●○

科研诚信和道德规范

2.1　科学中的价值观

　　科学家在调节科研工作和个人生活之间的平衡时，有选择研究课题的自由，并且有机会与各个领域的工作者合作，接触新的领域，其产生的新发现是令人兴奋的。同时，科学的飞速进步以及科学与社会关系的改变给科学界带来新的挑战，科研系统和科学家个人均面临着越来越大的压力。一方面，受过训练的研究人员数目的增加速度高于研究经费的增加速度；另一方面，研究工作变得更大、更复杂，需要越来越多的深入合作。

　　科学研究中存在着激烈竞争，伴随着无数的兴奋和挫折。科学知识的获得既是客观的研究获得，也是主观性很强的人为参与过程，不可避免地受到人的品行、价值观和局限性的影响，受到社会环境的影响。科学研究的成果既是属于科学家的个人成就，也同时依赖于全体科学家的共同努力，应属于公共的成果。科学知识的可靠性，来自科学家们的相互协作，必须以信任和自由为基础，也受到互相之间的约束。且新情况和新的相互关系层出不穷，研究工作受到的来自各方面的监督和管理也越来越严格。

　　本章内容所关注的问题主要涉及一般性错误、疏忽性错误和科学中不端行为之间的分界线，以及科学成就的荣誉应该如何分配。

2.2　实验技术与数据处理中的道德规范

2.2.1　实验方法的可靠性

　　实验方法的建立是为了客观证实科学发现。许多实验技术，包括著名的统计显著性测试、双盲试验等，都是力图将研究中个人主观偏见影响降到最小。研究人员必须正确掌握收集数据的可靠方法，规范操作，客观分析数据，才能得到有效数据。其他科学家也必须结合数据来源和获取数据的方法，才能判断数据的有效性。

2.2.2　数据的有效性

　　数据造假现象在全球科研范围内均有出现。英国爱丁堡大学从事学术不端行为研究的学者 Daniele Fanelli 发现，有 1.97% 科学家自己报告有数据造假行为，有 14.12% 的人知道同事有数据造假行为。医学领域和药理学领域是发生数据造假较多的领域。

　　以下仅举例说明几种常见的数据造假案例。

　　案例2-1：对图片的任意编辑。

　　Kenneth M. Yamada 于 2004 年在 *Journal of Cell Biology* 发表了题为："What's in a picture? The temptation of image manipulation" 的文章，文中详细介绍了多种通过对图片的任意编辑以取得想要结果的案例（*J. Cell Biol.* **2004**，166，11；已获授权许可）。

　　如图 2.1 所示，（a）组中原图的第 3 条带信号被删除。（b）组中原图的第 3 条带增加了信号。这是蛋白质印迹（western blot）最常见的造假方式。

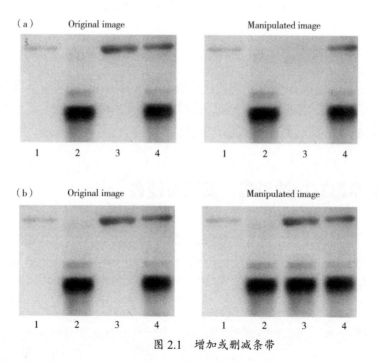

图 2.1　增加或删减条带

再如图 2.2 所示，通过调节原始数据对比度，突出实验组信号，减低对照组信号。这样的图像处理结果容易使读者对实验组做出错误判断。

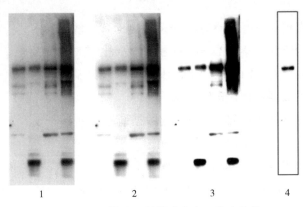

图 2.2　调节对比度以清除背景

案例2-2：一图多用。

同一个实验结果出现在不同的文章或文章中的不同实验中。2019 年 2 月 20 日 *Nature* 期刊撤回了 2018 年 9 月 5 日在发表的题为 "A homing system targets therapeutic T cells to brain cancer" 的研究论文。其中多处出现重复用图。

2.2.3　监督办法

目前包括 *Nature* 在内的众多杂志要求提供原始数据。人工智能技术的发展也为鉴别数据是否经过二次修改提供了强有力的工具。众多网站如 PubPeer 等也为监督数据的真伪提供了平台。

2.3　文章撰写中的引用、复述与抄袭

在科研工作中经常需要用到其他科学家的观点和工作基础，需要对他人的工作加以引用，但绝对不能抄袭。以下对引用他人工作成果的方式做一些说明。

2.3.1　直接引用

直接引用（Direct Quotation）是确切地再现别人所写过或说过的内

容，后面需要标注引用出处。直接引用的方式举例如下：

① As mentioned by Tom [Ref]…

② Tom [Ref] said that…

③ As Tom [Ref] says…

④ It's said by Tom [Ref] that…

2.3.2　复述

复述（Citation）是用自己的话重现别人所表达过的意思，是经过自己二次加工的，而不是直接重复原文，通常是用来支持自己的论点，也需要标注引用出处。复述的方式举例如下：

① Tom agreed that…[Ref]

② Tom have demonstrated that…[Ref]

③ It's generally accepted that…[Ref]

2.3.3　抄袭

按照哈佛大学网络公布的指引，抄袭（Plagiarism）通常包括以下 6 种类型。

（1）原文抄袭

直接重复原文而不标注原作者名。一些比较权威的查抄袭软件，诸如Turnitin、Crosscheck、iThenticate 等，有的判定连续 6 个单词和原文一样就属于抄袭。许多杂志社规定：包括绪论、方法、材料、测试方法及通讯地址在内，和之前已报道的所有文章相比重复率不得超过 20%，单篇重复率不得超过 5%。

（2）原作者标注缺失

在段落中某几句话借鉴了多篇文章，只对部分内容进行引文标注也属于抄袭。必须对文章中所有借鉴别人文章的语句进行标注，就算改写原话也需要进行标注。也可以加入自己的理解和进行总结式分析拓展，例如近期研究的一些不足之处等，这里可以不做标注。但前提是要有自己提炼的观点。

（3）不充分的复述

标注了原出处，但是对原文语句的改写不充分。例如只改写其中几个单词，查抄袭软件也是很容易查出来的。

（4）对原文进行了修改，但是没有标注原作者

当一个段落已经引用很多文章的时候，不想再连续标注；或者引用了同一篇文章中很多描述，无法取舍。这个时候，最好的办法就是只引用最经典的部分，或是原文中最重要的1～2句话。在论文写作中也应当注意引用文献的数量。引用文献数量太少，可能会出现调研不充分的情况；引用文献数量太多，又可能会给人一种无新意，只是改写的错觉。

（5）不标注原作者直接引用

对引用部分加上双引号，但是没有标注原作者也属于抄袭的一种。虽然有的同学认为双引号就是复述的意思，但是若不标注原作者，当读者想找原文时是检索找不到的。对于一些非正规的出处（如说非正式出版物、微博、毕业论文等），期刊一般都会有规范的引用格式要求。同时对于专业论文，力求引用出处的可靠性，尽量减少使用非正规出处引用。

（6）使用未公布的材料

使用未公开的不属于自己的材料，诸如同学的作业、未发表的文章、审稿中的文章和申请书等，都属于抄袭行为。在国外的许多大学，如果你抄袭同学的作业，严重的会面临退学处分。

2.3.4　一稿多投

论文的一稿多投是指同一作者或不同作者，在期刊编辑和审稿人不知情的情况下，已经或试图在多种期刊同时或相继发表内容相同或相近的论文，该种现象又被称为重复发表或自我剽窃。同一个工作投到不同杂志并发表，哪怕是同一个作者，都属于学术不端。将英文文章翻译成中文并二次发表也属于学术不端。

总的来说，相同研究成果的重复发表出现的情况较少，更常见的是作者就某个较大的课题陆续发表多篇论文。如果所涉及资料没有重复且每篇论文所讨论的问题各不相同，这种做法是可以接受的；但如果大量实验设计都相同，并存在同一批实验结果在不同杂志上多次使用，则可以定义为一稿多投。

一稿多投不仅仅是一个道德问题，更是法律禁止的行为。

2.4　学术造假的后果

学术造假对个人、集体、学术界，甚至是整个社会的发展都会带来严重的影响。

案例2-3：

2002 年春天，美国某大学教授 K 收到了一封匿名电子邮件，告知她的一篇论文被印度某大学校长 L 剽窃了。K 又听说该大学某主任 H 由于调查这桩剽窃案而丢掉工作，于是 K 起草了一封给印度总统的信件，信件中写道："如果印度科学的这个崇高的声誉被少数几个剽窃者所败坏，那真是太可惜了。"这封信通过媒体报道引起了总统关注，经过立案调查，L 论文剽窃案成立。2003 年 2 月，L 被印度政府撤了大学校长的职务。

在该案例中，剽窃者丧失了科研诚信，最终丢掉了工作，受到了来自社会各界的谴责。

案例2-4：

美国某大学一位科研人员，2008 年的时候发现兔子体内可以产生艾滋病病毒抗体，当时被学术界认为是重大科研成果。但实际上，他错误地将含有抗体的人血注入兔子血液中，从而导致实验结果看似是兔子体内产生抗体。当时他已经发现了错误，但是隐瞒不报，而且继续造假，直到其他研究人员揭穿了这场骗局。最终，该科研人员因为伪造研究数据、提交不实报告等重罪被起诉，获刑 5 年，罚款 720 万美元，出狱后还要接受 3 年的监外管制。

在该案例中，造假者不仅丢掉了工作，还受到了刑事处罚。

案例2-5：

韩国首尔大学教授 H 于 2004 年和 2005 年先后领导研究团队在 *Science* 杂志上发表论文，宣布成功克隆人类胚胎干细胞和患者匹配型干细胞，并陆续从韩国的一些财团、金融机构及政府领取了大量研究经费。2005 年年底，有关教授 H 干细胞学术造假的丑闻逐步被揭露。首尔大学经调查最终认定 H 学术造假，并宣布解除他的教授职务，韩国政府也取消了授予他的称号。韩国检察部门 2006 年 5 月对 H 提起诉讼，后期又对 H 提出诈骗、侵吞研究经费和非法买卖人体卵子违反《生命伦理法》等指控，要求法院判处其有期徒刑 4 年。

在该案例中，造假者严重浪费了来自社会各界的人力和资金资源，有的研究项目甚至可能进入临床，阻碍医学领域发展。最终造假者不仅被撤销一切称号及职位，并且被法院起诉。

2.5　成果的公开和发表

科研过程中时常会遇到利益相冲突的情况。例如：

① 研究人员收到的需要其评议的稿件，与他所做的工作相似，并领先一步；

② 已经完成的成果很可能会引起重大关注，但由于受到某项有限制的基金资助，不允许发表；

③ 几个课题组合作，发表的内容涉及其中某个课题组不愿公开的部分；

④ 企业资助的研究，科学家想尽快发表结果，而企业资助者想把结果保密，至少暂时保密；

⑤ 对于军事敏感性研究，公开发表研究结果也许是不可能的，而科学家迫切需要让同行认可其工作。

事实上，所有的科研单位都有相应的处理利益冲突的方法和措施、监督研究活动，以维护科研单位形象和科学诚信。许多科学杂志的编辑也建立了处理利益冲突的明确规章制度，在论文投稿阶段，研究人员需要告诉杂志编辑可能的利益冲突，让编辑决定采取什么方法处理。很多杂志社投稿时都需签署"Conflict of interest"。这些规章制度和措施维护着公众对科学诚实性的信心。

17 世纪，伦敦皇家学会秘书亨利·奥登伯格提出了现代投稿和审稿模式的雏形。在之前，许多科学家对其工作保密，他们担心一旦公布，别人会宣布优先权。亨利·奥登伯格提出对在学会的《哲学会刊》上发表过的文章的作者，由学会提供对于其优先权的官方证明，此外，他还将投稿文章送给能够判断其质量的专家审查。这些创新导致了现代科学杂志和同行评议制度的诞生。

社会共同约定的建立对于信息的有效共享并保护知识产权至关重要。

论文发表前，需要经过不同的审议。如果某人在别处使用了在投稿件中未发表的材料，这种行为就是盗窃知识产权。杂志社往往会让投稿者推荐5～6个审稿人并说明相应原因，同时给投稿者规避有冲突的审稿人的机会。当然杂志社并不会完全采纳推荐审稿人，而是由相应专业的编辑从该领域推荐审稿人。在工业界，科学研究工作的商业权利更多的是属于雇主而不是雇员，这些也都有相应的法律法规制定，如研究结果在发表或公开发布前是享有特权的，专利的申请也同样存在特权。论文发表后，科学家期望数据和研究材料与合格的科研工作者分享。

2.6　论文署名注意事项

在作者署名时也会出现荣誉分配问题。相对于过去，科学已成为一项需要更多合作的事业，越来越多的文章出现数个甚至数十个作者署名。合作使不同领域的研究人员相互交流，但同时增加了由署名引发问题的可能性。普遍认为，贡献最大的科学工作者位列第一；对课题的进行或文章的发表有着重要贡献的人，包括进行具体研究操作、获取数据的成员，解释数据的成员，进行论文撰写的成员，对论文进行科学指导的成员等，均为文章作者；通讯作者则是跟期刊编辑和评议人员沟通的成员，通常为导师或最重要的科研指导者。有些研究团体和杂志简单地按作者字母排名，从而避免署名问题，但在文章中要求详细列明每位作者的贡献。

通讯作者责任重大，需要确保所有作者都读过文章并认可文章的内容，并为其真实性和可靠性负责；需要确保文章发表后跟媒体、公众或者任何读者进行沟通。

而那些对文章有所贡献却没有列入作者署名的人员，如提供某种重要样品、提供资金资助、帮助润色论文等的人员，都应该放在致谢里。

坦率、公开地讨论荣誉分配非常重要。在研究工作刚开始时，明确任务分配；要发表论文时，所有合作者都要明确署名准则。现在很多杂志要求，投稿的原文和随后的修改稿，都要附有全部作者署名同意的信件。

需要明确的是，作者的排名不仅是一种荣誉，更是一种责任。当一篇论文中被发现含有错误，除非在脚注或论文中明确标明不同部分由不同作者负责，否则论文的所有署名作者必须全部承担责任。

2.7　总结

　　论文的发表呈现的是阶段性的工作成果。在这个意义上，所有的科学成果都可能被推翻。同时，科学家并没有无限的工作时间或无限的资源，也会无意识地犯错误。当这类错误被发现时，需要尽快在含有错误信息的同一杂志上承认错误。及时地、公开地承认错误会受到理解和尊重；而由于私心放任错误，甚至故意制造错误，则是非常恶劣的行为。科学家不应该以任何理由违反科研诚信和道德规范。

课后练习与讨论

1. 哪些行为属于学术不端？是什么导致了这些行为的产生？如何合理有效地制止这些行为？请针对各种情况提出自己的建议。
2. 若遇到学术不端事件，我们应该如何面对及正确处理？
3. 文章署名的顺序及注意事项有哪些？
4. 讨论以下案例。

　　在读研究生 M 参加了一个系里的讨论会，参加者以学生、博士后和教员为主。一个教员介绍了他的工作，M 发现自己研究的技术可以解决教员工作过程中遇到的问题，大力推动研究的进行，但 M 导师的研究方向与该教员的研究方向非常接近。请思考下列问题：

　　① M 是否应该在研讨会上介绍自己工作？应该怎么介绍？
　　② M 是否应该和导师讨论处理办法？是否应该和这位教员讨论课题？
　　③ 相较于传统的公开和资源共享，现代科学的数据、材料的共享面临哪些问题？有什么解决方案？

第 3 章 ●○

标题

3.1   标题及其重要性

标题是科技论文的纲要，需要以最准确、最简明的词语反映论文中重要发现的逻辑组合。对标题的每一个字和词语都需要认真斟酌，用最少的词语准确而有效地反映论文的内容。适宜的标题能够鲜明地揭示主题，体现出文章的中心内容，不要让读者去猜测题目的含义。另外，科学论文的标题必须具有自明性，可以自我解释。随着社会的发展，论文数量呈现不断增长的趋势。一个好的标题能提高读者对论文的注意力，激发读者的好奇心，进而吸引读者去阅读论文的主体内容。从以下两个例句可以说明文题的不同含义。

例如，"A Pharmacy Lab Report"（药剂学实验室报告），作为一篇论文的标题，它没有告诉读者任何信息，极不可取，充其量只能是一个栏目的标题。而"Effects of Polymer Concentration and Degree of Polymerization on Loading Capability of Microspheres"是一个较好的、较为全面的、能自我解释的题目。从表 3-1 中可以看出，这个题目十分准确地说明研究者所完成的 3 件事（即给予读者的信息）。

※ 表 3-1   不同标题给予读者不同的信息

序号	不同的标题	给予读者的信息
（1）	Effects of Polymer Concentration and Degree of Polymerization on Loading Capability of Microspheres	（1）The factors that were manipulated（polymer concentration and degree of polymerization） （2）The parameter that was measured（loading capability） （3）The specific object that was studied（microspheres）
（2）	Effects of Polymer Concentration and Degree of Polymerization on Microspheres	（1）The factors that were manipulated（polymer concentration and degree of polymerization） （2）No information about the measuring parameters （3）The specific object that was studied（microspheres）
（3）	Effects of Specific Factors on Loading Capability of Microspheres	（1）No information about the factors that were manipulated （2）The parameter that was measured（loading capability） （3）The specific object that was studied（microspheres）
（4）	Effects of Polymer Concentration and Degree of Polymerization on Loading Capability	（1）The factors that were manipulated（polymer concentration and degree of polymerization） （2）The parameter that was measured（loading capability） （3）No information about the specific object that was studied

改变一下标题，其含义就会发生明显的变化。如表 3-1（2）所示，假如

把标题改为 "Effects of Polymer Concentration and Degree of Polymerization on Microspheres"，那么读者就会猜测研究的测定指标是什么，是包封率、释药速率还是其他什么指标。如果把标题变换一下，改为表 3-1（3）所示 "Effects of Specific Factors on Loading Capability of Microspheres"，看到这一题目，读者立即会提出问题：什么特定的影响因素？影响因素包含了太广泛的内容，读者并不了解研究的影响因素到底是什么。如果把标题改为表 3-1（4）所示 "Effects of Polymer Concentration and Degree of Polymerization on Loading Capability"，对于这个标题，读者则无法知道研究者的研究对象是什么。这无形之中就会强迫读者去猜想或去阅读论文的部分内容，才能得到答案。故表 3-1 中（2）、（3）、（4）的 3 种情况，都属于包含信息不全、不能够自我解释的题目，缺乏自明性。

如果不是一种影响因素，而是多种（两种以上）因素时，题目中不宜将这些因素一一列出，而泛指 "影响因素" 即可。将标题改为 "Effects of Several Factors on Loading Capability of Microspheres"，似乎更为恰当。同样的道理，如果研究对象不是一个而是三到五个，不需要把所有研究对象的名字都列在标题中。在生物、医学科技论文的标题中，一般都会说明研究对象。如果研究对象是一种动物，特别是比较特殊的动物，应该呈现在题目中。如 "Anti-diabetic effect of American ginseng berry extracts on *ob/ob* mice"（"*ob/ob* mice" 即为特定的肥胖鼠的缩写）。假如研究中使用的是多种动物，不可能把全部动物名一一列出，这时可只让 "动物" 一词出现在标题中。而在更多的情况下，文题中常使用 "体内实验" 一词，即 "*in vivo*"。例如，"Effects of Notoginseng Extracts on Anticancer Property *in vivo*"。与 "体外实验" 相对应的就是 "体外实验"，即 "*in vitro*"。例如 "Antitumor Effect of American Ginseng Extracts on Human Colorectal Cancer Cell Lines *in vitro*"。不过需要注意的是，多数专业的 SCI 期刊要求 "*in vivo*" 和 "*in vitro*" 均为斜体。

3.2 标题结构

3.2.1 标题结构及词的顺序

英文论文标题多以短语为主要形式，尤以名词短语（noun phrase）最为常见，即标题基本上由一个或几个名词或名词短语加上其前置和（或）后置定语构成。

例 3-1：Oncolytic Virotherapy Promotes Intratumoral T Cell Infiltration and Improves Anti-PD-1 Immunotherapy.

例 3-2：Chemoresistance Evolution in Triple-Negative Breast Cancer Delineated by Single-Cell Sequencing.

例 3-3：Crystal Structure of the Human Cannabinoid Receptor CB1.

例 3-4：A Vulnerability of a Subset of Colon Cancers with Potential Clinical Utility.

在例 3-1 中，"Oncolytic Virotherapy"（溶瘤病毒治疗）是主要的名词短语作中心词，"Intratumoral T Cell Infiltration"（肿瘤内 T 细胞浸润）和"Improves Anti-PD-1 Immunotherapy"（改善 Anti-PD-1 免疫疗法）则为两个前置词后置定语，分别修饰、说明这种溶瘤病毒治疗的作用对象，以及能够取得怎样的效果。对于例 3-2 来说，中心词"Chemoresistance Evolution"（化疗耐药进化）是一个名词短语，"in Triple-Negative Breast Cancer"和"Delineated by Single-Cell Sequencing"也是两个前置词后置定语，用来修饰中心词"化疗耐药进化"，说明是针对什么疾病以及如何揭示的"化疗耐药进化"。其他两组例句也大同小异，都有自己主要的名词短语作中心及与其配合的前置词后置定语。

需要注意的是，短语型标题首先应该确定其中心词，而后再进行前后修饰，改变中心词有可能改变题意。标题中，各个词的顺序也很重要，词序不当，也会导致题意表达不准。

3.2.2 其他形式标题

（1）陈述句标题

从统计得知，使用陈述句作标题的比例不高。因为标题主要起标示作用，而陈述句容易使标题具有判断性的语义。况且陈述句不够精练和醒目，重点不突出。使用动词的标题，也就是使用句子作标题的比例较低。因此，应尽量减少使用句子作为标题。

如果十分必要的话，也不排除使用陈述句作标题。用完整句子作标题的文章，不仅出现在一般性的研究论文中，也出现在特殊的生物、医药学科技研究论文中。以下列举了 3 个标题作为例子，仅供参考。

例 3-5：Membrane Microdomain Disassembly Inhibits MRSA Antibiotic Resistance.

例 3-6：ATPase-Modulated Stress Granules Contain a Diverse Proteome and Substructure.

例 3-7：Cell-to-Cell Variation in p53 Dynamics Leads to Fractional Killing.

（2）疑问句标题

少数情况下，诸如评述性、综述性、驳斥性等类型的论文文题，也不排除使用疑问句作标题，因为疑问句具有较强的探讨性语气，也具有一定吸引力。相对而言，疑问句比较容易引起读者兴趣。以下选取了 5 个疑问句标题作为参考例句。

例 3-8：Dipeptidyl Peptidase-4 Inhibitors: Applications in Innate Immunity？

例 3-9：How Much Longer Will We Put up with $100,000 Cancer Drugs？

例 3-10：Is Ginseng Free from Adverse Effects？

例 3-11：Does "Non-interfacial lipids" Affect the Activity of Cytochrome Oxidase？

例 3-12：Animal Versus Human Oral Drug Bioavailability：Do They Correlate？

3.3　标题的字词数

3.3.1　选择标题字词数的标准

标题中用多少词最为合适，无统一规定。根据内容需要，建议使用 10～12 个词的英文标题，对于中文标题一般不超过 20 字。标题字词数的多少，应该取决于能否全面地表达论文的真正含义。标题过短显得过于简单化，提供的信息量不足，且不易表达完整的含义；而标题过长，显得累赘、冗长。应尽量用最少的字词来表达尽可能清楚而明确的内容。回顾表 3-1 中的第一个句子共 13 个词，能比较全面地阐明论文的意义。而标题 (2)、(3)、(4)，虽然少了几个词，但不能表达完整的含义。

3.3.2 "副标题"的使用

如果在命题时需要使用较多的字词才能表达完整而确切的意思，可使用"副标题"减少"主标题"的字词数。以下情况更适合采用"副标题"，例如：

① "主标题"语意未尽，用"副标题"补充说明论文的特定内容；

② 分阶段的研究结果，在同一"主标题"的情况下，用不同的"副标题"指出其特定内容，或完成了一系列研究工作，需要用几篇论文报道；

③ 其他有必要用"副标题"作为引申或说明的情况。

"副标题"使用得当，可使整个标题层次更为分明，含义更为清晰。以下 3 个例句可供参考。

例 3-13：Designer protein delivery: From natural to engineered affinity-controlled release systems.

例 3-14：Lisuride, a dopamine receptor agonist with 5-HT$_{2B}$ receptor antagonist properties: absence of cardiac valvulopathy adverse drug reaction reports supports the concept of a crucial role for 5-HT$_{2B}$ receptor agonism in cardiac valvular fibrosis.

例 3-15：Honokiol nanosuspensions: preparation, *in vitro* and *in vivo* evaluation.

3.3.3 标题中的冠词

在早期的科技论文标题中，冠词"the"用得较多。近些年冠词的使用趋向于简化，凡可用可不用的冠词在标题中均可省略不用。

例 3-16：The effects of three preparation technologies on the oral bioavailability of berberine α-hydroxy β-decanoylethyl sulfonate.

例 3-17：The inhibition effects of Pt（Ⅳ）on proliferation of breast cancer cells.

以上两个例句中的冠词"the"均在可用可不用之列，因此均可省略不用。题目不一定是句子，不需要完全符合英语句法要求，对冠词的处理应以简化为原则。

3.4 标题中英文字母的大小写

不同的期刊对标题中英文字母的大小写有不同的要求。纵观国际上的科技杂志，标题字母的大小写不外乎以下 3 种格式。

（1）全部字母大写

在标题中，不分词类也不论单词的大小，全部字母一律大写。目前使用这种格式的杂志逐渐减少。

例 3-18：DISSOLUTION SYSTEMS FOR CHLORAMPHENICOL TABLET BIOAVAILABILITY.

例 3-19：MICROENCAPSULATION AND CONTROLLED RELEASE OF INSULIN FROM POLYLACTIC ACID MICROCAPSULES.

（2）每个词的首字母大写

在标题中，每个词的首字母大写，但 3 或 4 个字母以下的冠词、连词、介词等小词全部小写。这是一种较为简化的书写格式。

例 3-20：Structure of the Nanobody-Stabilized Active State of the Kappa Opioid Receptor.

例 3-21：Manufacturing Process of Microcapsules for Autonomic Damage Repair of Polymeric Composites.

（3）第一个词的首字母大写

在标题中，只有第一个词的首字母大写，其他词的字母均小写。当然，缩写词及专有名词经常需要大写。这是一种更为简化的格式。

例 3-22：Drug delivery systems：Entering the mainstream.

例 3-23：Liposomes as "smart" pharmaceutical nanocarriers.

从目前的情况看，第一种格式（全部字母都大写）用得越来越少；第二种格式（每个词的首字母大写）用得较多；而第三种格式（标题的第一个词的首字母大写）的使用有逐年增多的趋势。从题目字母大小写的变化及标题中冠词使用的变化，可以看出人们对科技论文撰写的倾向性变化：简化写作的趋向。写作需要简化，出版更需要简化。

3.5　命题中的禁忌

在汉语中，人们习惯使用"……的研究""……的实验研究""……的实验观察""……的初步研究""试论……的……""……的考略""……的浅论""……的初探"等命题格式，但在撰写英文论文时，应尽量加以避免。实际上，无论是"实验"，还是"观察"，或是"研究"等，都是完全无用的词，应该避免使用这些"废词"（waste word）。因为论文本身就是实验、观察、研究，无需在题目中进行强调。因此"Studies on...""An investigation of..."或"Experimental observation of..."等词语不应在英文标题中出现。

例 3-24：The study of lipid-lowering effect of Atorvastatin Calcium microspheres on hyperlipidemia model of rats.（阿托伐他汀钙微球对高脂血症模型大鼠降脂作用的研究）

例 3-25：The experimental study of effect of Atorvastatin Calcium microspheres on hyperlipidemia model of rats.（阿托伐他汀钙微球对高脂血症模型大鼠作用的实验研究）

上述两个标题都应该属于不易被接受的命题格式。可被接受的命题应该是把能够去除的"废词"及"垃圾词"全部丢掉，同时把可用可不用的冠词也一并删除，形成一个简明而清晰的标题。

例 3-26：Lipid-lowering effect of Atorvastatin Calcium microspheres on hyperlipidemia model of rats.（阿托伐他汀钙微球对高脂血症模型大鼠的降脂作用）

如例 3-26 所示，尽量减少缩略词的使用，提高论文标题的自明性，避免不必要的麻烦。只有得到公认的缩略词，才可用于标题中。为了方便阅读和理解，在论文第一次出现科技语时，需要加以解释、说明或定义。在标题中应完全避免使用阿拉伯数字。如非用不可，则应把数字改为英文。

例 3-27："121 cases"应改为"One hundred and twenty-one cases"。

例 3-28："76 rabbits…"应改为"Seventy six rabbits..."。

3.6 标题中常用的英语词组和表达方式

标题中常见的错误有省略不当、介词使用不当、并列关系使用不当、用词不当、句子混乱、标题冗长、文题不符、重复和歧义等。为避免这些错误的发生，本节将标题中常用的几种英语词组及表达方式介绍如下。

3.6.1 一般特征的研究

例 3-29：Characterization and evaluation of functional polymer microspheres with core-shell structure.

例 3-30：Structure of a DNA glycosylase searching for lesions.

例 3-31：Structural stability of Cytochrome C in Egg Phosphatidylcholine liposomes.

例 3-32：Changes in structure of BPP after interaction with Cl/PC liposomes.

3.6.2 A对B的作用 （Effect of A on B）

例 3-33：Effect of insulin-loaded PLGA microspheres on osteogenesis around implants of type 2 diabetic rats.

例 3-34：Effect of curcumin microcapsules on serum lipids and liver pathology of hyperlipidemic rats.

例 3-35：Effect of hyperbranched polymer on properties of polypropylene/sisal fiber composites.

3.6.3 A与B的关系

例 3-36：The relation between courses of lipo-PGE1 treatment and blood-supply improvement in diabetic foot patients.

例 3-37：The relationship between the dissolubility of oral solid preparation and the body bioavailability.

例 3-38：The relationship between bioavailability and dissolution profile of cefalexin tablets *in vitro*.

例 3-39：The interrelationship between the structure and characterization of alginate microspheres.

3.7　文章标题示例

这里提供标题字词数适中的、不同类型的 13 篇文章标题，供命题时参考。

① Asparagine bioavailability governs metastasis in a model of breast cancer.

② Antibacterial Nucleoside-Analog Inhibitor of Bacterial RNA Polymerase.

③ Spinal cord injury alters cardiac electrophysiology and increases the susceptibility to ventricular arrhythmias.

④ Common features of enveloped viruses and implications for immunogen design for next-generation vaccines.

⑤ Modification of cellular communication by gene transfer.

⑥ Visualization of membrane pore in live cells reveals a dynamic-pore theory governing fusion and endocytosis.

⑦ Molecular correlates of repolarization alternans in cardiac myocytes.

⑧ High efficiency activation of L-type Ca^{2+} current by 5-HT in human atrial myocytes.

⑨ Serum antibody responses after intradermal vaccination against influenza.

⑩ Synthesis of polymeric microcapsule arrays and their use for enzyme immobilization.

⑪ PEBP1 wardens ferroptosis by enabling lipoxygenase generation of lipid death signals.

⑫ Effects of dietary supplements on coagulation and platelet function.

⑬ Anti-diabetic effect of American ginseng may not be linked to antioxidant activity: Comparison between American ginseng and Scutellaria baicalensis using an *ob/ob* mice model.

课后练习与讨论

1. 什么样的标题才是有意义的标题？撰写标题需注意哪些要点？
2. 一篇文章的标题拟定后，如何评估其是否恰当。
3. 根据本章的内容，选定几篇药学专业论文，分析其中标题的内容和结构。
4. 选取几篇药学专业论文，根据本章所述标题命名的原则试拟标题，并与原文标题进行比较分析。

第 4 章 ●○

摘要

4.1　摘要的作用与主要内容

摘要（Abstract）是对论文的内容不加注释和评论的简短陈述，是一种高度概括的文体，需要简明扼要地说明研究工作的目的、研究方法和最终结论等，是一篇具有独立性和完整性的短文。摘要是一篇论文的缩影，也是论文中最重要的一部分。一篇正式的英文论文应当附有论文摘要，非英语论文应附有英文摘要。不同期刊对"摘要"的字数有不同的要求。从 80 个字到 400 个字不等，绝大多数为 150～250 个字。

摘要是以提供论文内容概要为目的，简单而确切地记述论文的主要内容，让读者获得必要的信息。摘要应具有独立性和自明性，并且含有与论文全文同等的主要信息，即使读者在没有阅读全文的情况下，也可得到应有的信息。由于国际学术交流的需要，英文摘要在中文科技论文中具有特殊的作用。随着中国科学技术水平的快速发展和国际地位的不断提高，世界各国都会订阅一些高水平的中文杂志。英文摘要、图表的英文注释可以帮助国外读者理解论文的主要研究内容。

结构式摘要广泛应用到生物、医药学基础研究及临床的各个学科领域。所谓结构式摘要就是要求作者按照一定的结构模式撰写摘要。一般要求结构式摘要的杂志都有既定的模式。生物医学科技论文的一般结构模式为：背景（background）；目的（objective/purpose）；方法（methods）；结果（results/findings）；结论（conclusions）。

4.2　几种类型的摘要模式

这里展示了几种不同类型的英语摘要模式。需要说明的是，以下所要讨论的例 4-1 至例 4-3 摘自不同杂志，因此，在形式上存在着一定的差异。

例 4-1　*Cell* **2018**, 172, 55.（已获授权许可）

Title: Structure of the Nanobody-Stabilized Active State of the Kappa Opioid Receptor

Abstract: The kappa-opioid receptor (KOP) mediates the actions of opioids with hallucinogenic, dysphoric, and analgesic activities. The design of KOP analgesics devoid of hallucinatory and dysphoric effects has been hindered by an incomplete structural and mechanistic understanding of KOP agonist actions. Here, we provide a crystal structure of human KOP in complex with the potent epoxymorphinan opioid agonist MP1104 and an activestate-stabilizing nanobody. Comparisons between inactive-and active-state opioid receptor structures reveal substantial conformational changes in the binding pocket and intracellular and extracellular regions. Extensive structural analysis and experimental validation illuminate key residues that propagate larger-scale structural rearrangements and transducer binding that, collectively, elucidate the structural determinants of KOP pharmacology, function, and biased signaling. These molecular insights promise to accelerate the structure-guided design of safer and more effective k-opioid receptor therapeutics.

例 4-2 *Acta Pharm. Sim.* **2003**,38,133.（已获授权许可）

Title: Preparation of cisplatin multivesicular liposomes and release of cisplatin from the liposomes *in vitro*

Abstract:

AIM: To prepare cisplatin multivesicular liposomes with high encapsulation efficiency and sustained-release character, and compare the release characteristics with conventional liposomes prepared by reverse-phase evaporation method.

METHODS: Cisplatin multivesicular liposomes were prepared using multiple emulsion method. The concentrations of cisplatin and lipids in the liposomes were measured by flameless atomic absorbance spectroscopy (FAAS) and phosphalipid enzyme reagent method, respectively. The encapsulation efficiency, size and release of the cisplatin from the liposomes were studied *in vitro*.

RESULTS: The mean diameter of cisplatin multivesicular liposomes was (16.6 +/−1.0) micron. The encapsulation efficiency of cisplatin was more than 80%. The release profile in vitro fitted with a first-order equation. The releasing $t_{1/2}$ of cisplatin multivesicular liposomes is 37.7 h, which is 8.4 that of conventional liposomes. Co-membrane stabilizer has remarkable stabilizing effect on the multivesicular liposomal membrane confirmed by differential scattering calorimetry (DSC).

CONCLUSION: The cisplatin multivesicular liposomes showed high encapsulation efficiency and sustained-release character.

例4-3　*Cell* **2003**，485，89.（已获授权许可）

Title: Prediction of drug bioavailability based on molecular structure

Abstract: Oral dosing is the most common method of drug administration, and final plasma concentrations of the drug depend upon its bioavailability. In the current study, a quantitative structure-pharmacokinetic relationship (QSPR) was developed for a diverse range of compounds to allow prediction of drug bioavailability. Bioavailability data for 169 compounds was taken from the literature, and from the molecular structures 94 theoretical descriptors were generated. Stepwise regression was employed to develop a regression equation based on 159 training compounds, and predictive ability was tested on 10 compounds reserved for that purpose. The final regression equation included eight descriptors that represented electronic, steric, hydrophobic and constituent parameters of the drug molecules, all of which could be related to solubility and partitioning properties. Predicted bioavailability for the training set agreed more closely for drugs exhibiting mid-range literature bioavailability values. A correlation of 0.72 was achieved for test set bioavailability predictions when compared with literature values. The structure-pharmacokinetic relationship developed in the current study highlighted solubility and partitioning characteristics that may be useful in designing drugs with appropriate bioavailability.

4.3　摘要的结构分析

　　不同类型的摘要有不同的结构要求。这里主要分析生物医学科技论文中"摘要"的结构，即为前述"结构式摘要"的基本结构。由于不同杂志对

"摘要"的格式有不同的要求，因此，在"摘要"的结构上也有明显的差别。在这一节里，将重点分析 4.2 节几种典型的摘要格式中的 3 个例子。

（1）"例 4-1"的分析

例 4-1 这篇摘要基本上属于结构式摘要，主要包括原理（该项研究的背景知识）、实验目的、新的发现（通常包括采用的实验手段）和结论，共由 6 个句子组成。前两个句子指出了这项研究的背景资料："The kappa-opioid receptor（KOP）mediates the actions of opioids with hallucinogenic, dysphoric, and analgesic activities. The design of KOP analgesics devoid of hallucinatory and dysphoric effects has been hindered by an incomplete structural and mechanistic understanding of KOP agonist actions."通过这两个句子，读者可以了解到 KOP（κ 阿片受体）的作用。此外，作者指出了目前尚未解决的一个问题，即"设计没有致幻和烦躁作用的 KOP 镇痛药受到了阻碍"，这也阐明了这项研究的目的——设计更安全有效的 KOP 镇痛药。接下来的 3 个句子（第 3～5 句）是摘要中的发现和结果部分，也包括采取的研究方法。第 6 个句子，"These molecular insights promise to accelerate the structure-guided design of safer and more effective κ-opioid receptor therapeutics."阐明了这项研究的意义，并且与上面所提到的研究目的相呼应。

（2）"例 4-2"的分析

例 4-2 这篇摘要也是一种典型的结构式摘要。其结构包括 4 个部分：background（或 purpose、aim、objective）、methods、results 和 conclusions。在第 1 部分"AIM"（目的）中，作者只用了 1 个句子来阐明研究目的。第 2 部分"METHODS"（方法）中，作者用了 3 个句子来描述他们在研究中所使用的方法。在第 3 部分"RESULTS"（结果）中，作者使用了 5 个句子来阐述所得的结果，重在说明粒径、包封率、体外释放度等参数。而在最后的"CONCLUSION"（结论）中，作者也只用了 1 个句子概述了研究的结论。

（3）"例 4-3"的分析

例 4-3 这篇摘要是一篇简明扼要的摘要，共由 8 句话组成。除了开头和结尾，作者各用一句话分别介绍相关背景和概括研究的意义外，中间 6 句话都用来描述研究的方法和结果。这一方面说明了摘要中方法和结果的重要性，另一方面也表现出作者对结果的重视程度。

除了为突出内容这一原因外，期刊的受众也在一定程度上决定了摘要需要集中笔墨在研究结果。摘要的主要目的是让广泛的读者群能认识到所报道内容的重要性及其概念上的进展，摘要内不应引用文献。专业期刊面向的主要读者群是从事与专业有关的科学家及学者，在背景材料方面，就只需要介绍与所报道的研究最相关的少量信息。

4.4　摘要中应避免的问题

摘要写作中应该注意避免以下问题：

① 应避免在摘要的第一句话重复使用标题或标题的一部分，避免与正文中的句子重复。

② 摘要中结果虽应重点介绍，但是，应把最新的、最重要的、最能说明问题的结果列出，放在几个句子中，避免过细的结果描述。同时应避免过于笼统、空洞无物的一般论述和结论。

③ 摘要是具有高度概括性的文体，要求篇幅尽量小，句子尽量少且完整。不谈或尽量少谈（最多用一句话）背景材料。

④ 摘要应该是纯文字叙述，避免使用插图、表格、化学结构式、数学公式及参考文献等。

⑤ 摘要应避免使用第二人称。前述举例的摘要都使用了第一人称，优点在于比较直截了当，把想法、研究结果和结论直言不讳地介绍给读者，更具有说服力。

⑥ 避免使用一些具有"投机性"的词汇，诸如"obviously""probably""certainly""undoubtedly"等。使用这些词汇只是一般的假设或猜测，并不能也无法证明这些观点。

4.5　摘要中的英语时态和语态

4.5.1　英语时态

在摘要中英语的时态变化较多，包括一般现在时、一般过去时、现在完成时等。一般过去时最为常见，特别是在结果中。一般来说，英语摘要中时态的运用也以简练为佳，常用一般现在时和一般过去时；少用现在完成时和过去完成时；现在进行时和过去进行时及其复合时态则基本不用。

（1）一般现在时

一般现在时用于说明研究目的、叙述研究内容、描述结果、得出结论、提出建议或讨论等。另外，凡涉及公认事实、自然规律、永恒真理等，也用一般现在时。

（2）一般过去时

一般过去时用于叙述过去某一时刻（时段）的结果和发现，以及某一研究过程（包括实验、调查、观察、医疗等过程）。在结果和（或）结论中用一般过去时是说明当时的情况。对规律性的事物则往往用一般现在时表达。

（3）现在完成时

现在完成时表明过程的延续性，虽然某事件或过程发生在过去，但强调对现实所产生的影响。也就是把过去发生的或过去已经完成的事情与现在联系起来。例4-4与例4-5为现在完成时的使用参考。

例4-4：However, developing selective deubiquitinase inhibitors has been challenging and no co-crystal structures have been solved with small-molecule inhibitors.

例4-5：Since the discovery by Ullmann and Bielecki in 1901，reductive dimerization（or homocoupling）of aryl halides has been extensively exploited for the generation of a range of biaryl-based functional molecules.

（4）过去完成时

过去完成时可用来表达过去某一时间以前已经完成的事情，或在过去的一个事情完成之前就已完成的另一个过去的行为。

4.5.2　英语语态

过去的论文，包括摘要多使用被动语态。强调被动语态的理由是生物医学科技论文主要是说明事实经过，至于是谁做的并不重要，也无需一一证明或介绍。被动语态可在主语部分集中较多的信息，起到信息前置、语义突出的效果。请参考例 4-6 和例 4-7。

例 4-6：Although efficacy with multiple viral vaccine platforms has been established in animals, no study has addressed protection during pregnancy.

例 4-7：By contrast，many proteins containing cleavable amino-terminal signal peptides were efficiently cotranslationally targeted in SRP's absence.

现在使用主动语态的论文摘要逐年增多。因为主动语态有助于文字表述清晰、简洁明快且表达有力，给人一种干净利落的感觉。请参考例 4-8 和例 4-9。

例 4-8：Our results suggest a simple model whereby ketamine quickly elevates mood by blocking NMDAR-dependent bursting activity of LHb neurons to disinhibit downstream monoaminergic reward centres, and provide a framework for developing new rapid-acting antidepressants.

例 4-9：Here we report the crystal structure of DRD2 in complex with the widely prescribed atypical antipsychotic drug risperidone.

4.6 摘要中常用的英语词组和表达方式

4.6.1 研究目的

简要陈述研究宗旨，说明研究要解决的问题，一般只用一句话来表达。常用英语词组为动词不定式，不同的研究目的用不同的不定式。例如：为研究——to study, to investigate；为观察——to observe；为探索——to explore；为评价——to evaluate；为证实、证明——to confirm, to demonstrate；为比较——to compare 等。

例 4-10：The purpose of this investigation was to develop a quantitative structure-bioavailability relationship (QSBR) model for drug discovery and development.

例 4-11：The aim of the present pilot study was to characterize the renal...

例 4-12： To compare the biocompatibility of the alginate-polylysine-alginate (APA) microcapsule and the alginate-chitosan-polyethyleneglycol (ACP) microcapsute which newly developed in our laboratory.

例 4-13：The purpose of this article is to review the history and classification of proteinase inhibitors.

例 4-14：To determine the effects on the structure formation of comminuted meat emulsions…

例 4-15：The purpose of this study was to test the hypothesis that inhibition of NCX with a newly developed selective NCX inhibitor（SEA0400）reduces TdP.

4.6.2 研究方法

摘要中的研究方法是指简明扼要地介绍研究途径、采用的材料、实验模型、实验范围及手段等。在摘要中，研究方法的介绍必须极为简要。在大部分情况下，只需说明方法的名称。摘要中常用的英语词组有："by means of""by using""by the use of""using...as..."等。

例 4-16：GNA-NLC was prepared by means of emulsion evaporation-low temperature solidification.

例 4-17：We screened similar to 800,000 random peptide sequences for antimicrobial function and identified thousands of active sequences by using SLAY.

例 4-18：We investigated the role of intracellular calcium cycling... using the perforated or ruptured patch clamp techniques...

例 4-19：Using the technique of microemulsion polymerization with nano-reactor, dysprosium ferrite/polyacrylamide magnetic composite microsphere was prepared by one-step method in a single inverse microemulsion.

例 4-20：We studied 53 patients with left ventricular ejection fraction（28±8）% and 18 control subjects. Monophasic APs were recorded in the right ventricle （$n=62$）and/or left ventricle（$n=9$）at 109 beats/min.

4.6.3 研究结果

摘要中的研究结果应包括本研究所获得的新资料、新数据等。这是摘要的根本所在，应该把主要结果介绍清楚。不少论文常习惯使用"that"从句表达实验结果。例如：

The results indicate that...

The data show that...

The results demonstrated that...

The data reveal that...

研究结果的写作范例如下。

例4-21：The result indicated that P9, with half-sequence ionic complement, may serve as a hydrophobic compounds carrier.

例4-22：Analysis of the effects of the treatment on stability, structural and rheological properties, and texture of the emulsions end products showed that addition of sodium caseinate and BPP caused a deterioration in textural...

例4-23：Disease-free survival in the capecitabine group was at least equivalent to that in the flurouracil-plus-Ieucovorin group (in the intention-to-teat analysis, $P < 0.001$ for the comparison of the upper limit of the hazard ratio with the noninferiority margin of 1.20). Capecitabine improved relapse-free survival (hazard ratio 0.86; 95 percent confidence interval, 0.74 to 0.99; $P = 0.05$) and was associate with significantly fewer adverse events than fluorouracil plus leucovorin ($P < 0.001$).

4.6.4　研究结论及其意义

根据实验结果，恰到好处地作出结论，并探讨可能的理论价值和实际意义，一般只需用一句话来表达。

研究结论及研究意义部分的写作范例如下。

例4-24：The result indicated that P9, with half-sequence ionic complement, may serve as a hydrophobic compounds carrier.

例4-25：Our tissue recombination assay provides an empirical test to examine the relationship of PIN to prostate carcinoma.

例4-26：Here we report the multistage antiplasmodial activity of the aspartic protease inhibitor hydroxyl-ethyl-amine-based scaffold compound 49c.

例4-27：In this context, we also report a convenient synthesis of T2O from T-2, providing access to high-specific-activity T2O. This protocol has been successfully applied to the high incorporation of deuterium and tritium in 18 drug molecules, which meet the requirements for use in ligand-binding assays and absorption, distribution, metabolism, and excretion studies.

例4-28：These results elucidate SRP's essential roles in maintaining the efficiency and specificity of protein targeting.

例4-29：These findings suggest that targeting of GPX4 may represent a therapeutic strategy to prevent acquired drug resistance.

课后练习与讨论

1. 文章的摘要应该起什么样的作用？它分为哪些类型？分别适用于什么样的论文？
2. 选择几篇药学专业论文，分析摘要的类型以及每句话在摘要中的作用。
3. 选取若干篇药学专业论文，精读后尝试撰写其摘要，并与原文的摘要进行比较分析。

第 5 章 •○

背景介绍

5.1　背景介绍的写作

5.1.1　背景介绍的要素

背景介绍（Introduction）也称"引言""简介"等，是论文正文的第一部分，也是对摘要的进一步扩展。Introduction 主要介绍与本研究相关的背景知识，以便读者更好地理解该论文解决了什么科学问题，其成果和发现的重要性，以及它们是如何促进和推动当前该领域向前发展的。通常来说，背景介绍必须包括六大要素：研究主题、学术重要性、文献调研、知识缺口、研究问题、研究成果及贡献。

（1）研究主题（Theme 或 Topic）

介绍研究主题有助于读者清晰地理解该论文研究的是什么，其写作要点包括：

① 避免使用技术行话；

② 不要从研究问题或假设开始引言部分；

③ 定义专业术语和概念。

（2）学术重要性（Academic Importance）

需要强调研究主题的学术和（或）应用价值，表明该研究值得进一步探讨。

（3）文献调研（Literature Review）

文献调研主要包含与主题相关的最重要和最新的研究成果，让读者对该领域的当前研究水平有比较清晰的了解，而不需要对整个领域写一个综合的回顾。

（4）知识缺口（Knowledge Gap）

知识缺口用于说明需要解决的具体知识缺口以及与文献中的不一致、有争议的问题。

（5）研究问题（Research Question）

研究问题主要用于说明：

① 本文的研究问题。

② 设定的研究目标。

③ 论文中所使用的方法和技术。

（6）研究成果及贡献（Results and Contributions）

虽然详细的研究成果会在接下来的"实验结果"和"讨论"部分进行更深入的阐述和探讨，但在背景介绍中，仍然需要用简短的方式，突出本研究的主要成果及贡献，以及该研究工作对所研究领域未来的影响。这有助于审稿人和读者在进一步阅读"实验结果"和"讨论"部分前对全文有一个宏观的了解。

5.1.2　背景介绍的写作范例

例5-1：背景介绍内容引自 *J. Med. Chem.* **2014**，57，8249.（已获授权许可，版权所有©2014，美国化学会）

（1）研究主题

The role of the epidermal growth factor receptor (EGFR) in non-small-cell lung cancer is well-known, and substantial therapeutic progress in the treatment of this disease has been made over the past 10 years through the exploitation of this insight. Inhibition of the kinase domain of EGFR and resultant oncogenic cell signaling disruption by small molecule inhibitors such as gefitinib 1 and erlotinib 2 (Figure 1) have been shown to be particularly beneficial in those patients carrying the so-called "sensitizing mutations" such as L858R and the exon-19 deletion.

（2）学术重要性

The subsequent identification of irreversible EGFR inhibitors such as dacomitinib 3 and afatinib 4 (Figure 1) that inhibit both mutants described above as well as the wild type receptor potentially offers therapeutic options for T790M positive patients.

（3）文献调研

Recently, both ourselves (compound 5, Figure 2) and others (*N*-[3-[5-chloro-2-

[[2-methoxy-4-(4-methylpiperazin-1-yl)-phenyl]amino]pyrimidin-4-yl]oxyphenyl] prop-2-enamide (WZ4002), 6, Gatekeeper Pharmaceuticals Inc.; *N*-[3-[[2-[[4-(4-acetylpiperazin-1-yl)-2-methoxyphenyl]amino]-5-chloropyrimidin4-yl]amino] phenyl]prop-2-enamide (CO-1686), 7, Clovis Oncology) have described efforts to identify mutant selective inhibitors that target both the sensitizing mutations and the T790M resistance mutation while also sparing the wild type form of the receptor, inhibition of which can lead to dose limiting toxicities including skin rash and diarrhea.

（4）知识缺口

However, the high wild-type potency and accompanying toxicities associated with such activity may well limit their utility in this setting.

（5）研究问题

Herein, we describe some of our work that has led to the identification of the clinical candidate AZD9291 (8).

（6）研究成果及贡献

a potent inhibitor of both sensitizing and double mutant (sensitizing and T790M resistance) forms of EGFR with selectivity over the wild type form (Figure 2).

例5-2：背景介绍内容引自 *Clin. Ther.* **2014**，36，128.（已获授权许可）

（1）研究主题

Spinal muscular atrophies (SMAs) are a group of hereditary autosomal recessive neuromuscular diseases that are characterized by the degeneration of motor neurons in the spinal cord and brainstem, resulting in progressive proximal muscle weakness, hyposthenia, and paralysis, which are usually symmetrical.

（2）学术重要性

The increased attention to early diagnosis and to several aspects of management of SMA has stimulated the development of clinical guidelines and standards of care.

（3）文献调研

SMA is the most frequent genetic cause of infant mortality, with an estimated incidence of 1 in 6000 to 1 in 10000 live births and a carrier frequency of 1 in 40 to 1 in 60. The classical form of the disorder is caused by a genetic mutation in the 5q11.2-q13.3 locus, which affects the survival motor neuron (SMN) gene and leads to the reduction of SMN protein. SMA is clinically conventionally classified into 4 phenotypes (Ⅰ, Ⅱ, Ⅲ, and Ⅳ) on the basis of age of onset and highest motor function achieved, with an additional phenotype (type 0) to describe the severe forms with an antenatal onset. Prognosis depends on the phenotypic severity, ranging from high mortality within the first year for SMA type I to no mortality for the chronic and later-onset forms.

（4）知识缺口

In the past decade, many promising new therapeutic approaches have been tested in clinical trials of patients with SMA but with limited or no success.

（5）研究问题

Consequently, the development of novel therapies in SMA now has strong academic, government, and industry involvement, in addition to the interest of several parental organizations and foundations.

（6）研究成果及贡献

The goal of the present article was to summarize the literature on the emerging molecular therapeutic approaches that are currently being investigated or planned to be tested in clinical trials of SMA (Figure 1).

例5-3：背景介绍内容引自 *J. Med. Chem.* **2010**, 53, 7202.（已获授权许可，版权所有©2010，美国化学会）

（1）研究主题

HCV is a plus strand RNA virus of the *Flaviviridea* family with a 9.6 kb genome encoding for 10 proteins: three structural proteins and seven nonstructural proteins. The nonstructural proteins, which include the NS5B RNA dependent RNA polymerase (RdRp), provide several attractive targets for the development of anti-HCV therapy. The HCV RdRp is part of a membrane associated replication complex that is composed of other viral proteins, viral RNA, and altered cellular membranes.

（2）学术重要性

The hepatitis C virus (HCV) presents a global health problem with approximately 180 million individuals infected worldwide with 80% of those progressing to chronic HCV infection. Of those chronically infected individuals, approximately 30% will develop liver cirrhosis and 10% will go on to develop hepatocellular carcinoma.

（3）文献调研

As in the case of other viral polymerases, two approaches have been pursued to identify small molecule HCV NS5B polymerase inhibitors. These approaches include the identification of nucleoside analogues that function as alternative substrate inhibitors that induce a chain termination event and non-nucleoside inhibitors that bind to allosteric sites on the polymerase leading to a nonfunctional enzyme.

（4）知识缺口

In addition, drug discontinuations may be high because of adverse side effects associated with the SOC treatment regimen. Consequently, the development of alternative treatment options is greatly needed. The search for novel therapies for the treatment of HCV infection has focused on the development of direct acting antiviral agents (DAAs).

（5）研究问题

However, even with the positive clinical attributes of 1, we were interested in investigating second generation agents with improved potency, enhanced pharmacokinetic properties (i.e., q.d. dosing), and the potential for generating high concentrations of the active triphosphate in the liver to enable low doses and potentially fixed-dose combinations of DAAs. To achieve this objective, we focused on *β-D-2′-deoxy-2′-α-F-2′-β-C*-methyluridine (5) (Figure 2).

（6）研究成果及贡献

Here we describe the discovery of phosphoramidate prodrugs of 2′-deoxy-2′-α-F-2′-β-C-methyluridine 5′-monophosphate and the selection of 14 and ultimately of its single isomer 51 as clinical development candidates.

5.2　文献调研的写作

5.2.1　文献调研的写作方法和技巧

文献调研是该论文立项的理论基础，并讨论该领域的当前研究进展。它包含了总结、批评、分析、综合、评估以及对信息的重新组织。文献调研是追溯该领域研究的进展，为读者，尤其是不熟悉该研究领域的读者提供一个较为全面的理论和知识框架。

撰写文献调研一般包括以下六个方面。

（1）文献调研内容选取的要点

① 定义论文中所有的关键概念和术语。

② 简要地讨论本研究和该领域研究的相关性。

③ 对之前该领域相关成果的既综合又聚焦的讨论。

④ 对本研究的立题和假设铺垫理论基础。

（2）文献调研的信息组织

文献调研不是简单地按照时间顺序进行文献总结，因此需要有条理地组织当前已有的知识。下面从三个方面来描述文献调研信息的组织：

① 定义：所有的概念和专业术语都要被定义，且最好是在其第一次出现后就马上定义。同时也要注意，不要直接从原论文中照搬过来，而要用自己的话描述。

② 属性或要素：对于相关的属性或要素进行总结，而不只是单单的罗列出来。

③ 对立的观点：应该清楚地解释对立观点的不同之处。

（3）文献调研的架构

文献调研的结构应该是富有逻辑的，每一部分之间都要密切联系起来。

① 首先从相关研究领域的宏观背景开始，然后聚焦到所要研究的具体问题上。

② 可以使用相关的示意图。

③ 对研究的重要概念进行比较。

④ 明确地定义专业术语和概念。

⑤ 提供对研究假设或动机的简要描述。

（4）文献调研的写作风格

① 文献调研应该易于阅读和理解。

② 文中首次出现的专业术语和概念应给予清晰明确的定义，避免不规范的缩写。

③ 制订一个清晰简洁的流程帮助读者理解，尤其是针对不熟悉该研究领域的审稿人和读者。

④ 仅需对研究内容相关的文献进行总结。

（5）说明当前结论有冲突或未解决的问题

通过比较两个研究的异同点，或者对之前的研究进行总结概括，发现一个有争议的、有问题的，或者未经科学检验的假设，或者在已有的研究中没有使用的方法，明确当前研究的不足。

（6）批评之前已报道的研究

在指出当前知识缺口的过程中，难免会批评已有的研究，需要注意的是，被批评的研究者很可能就是论文的审稿人，要考虑他们的感受。而且有时作者的批评可能是错误的，这会损害他们在这一领域的名声。以下的建议将有助于开展健康的学术批评：

① 永远不要使得批评成为对某篇文献或某项研究的个人攻击；

② 批评必须建立在客观公正的立场上，要有充分的理由；

③ 不要为了批评而批评，以过度地体现本论文研究的重要性和与众不同；

④ 咨询该领域的其他学者，以更好地评判该批评是否是有效的；

⑤ 批评时的写作用语要相对含蓄，要留有余地。除非你已经在该领域内有极高的学术地位。

5.2.2 文献调研的写作建议

关于撰写文献调研的一些建议：

① 从一般到具体。把生活中的问题和文献相联系，然后引到作者的研究。

② 吸引读者的注意。回答下面的问题："你做了什么？""为什么我要关心？"

③ 清晰地呈现你的问题和解决方案、你的疑问和你的实验设计、你之前和现在所做的实验之间的联系。

④ 尽可能多地使用主动语态。

5.2.3 文献调研的常用句型

5.2.3.1 描述所要研究的问题

（1）建立所要研究主题的重要性

① Kinases have been intensively investigated as drug targets for the past 30 years ...

② The challenge that this presents for drug discovery is highlighted by the fact that…

③ 16-memberd macrolides is an important kind of bacteriostat drug…

④ Significant challenges in obtaining sufficient systemic exposure...

（2）从强调时间开始

① The early 2000s brought a new age in the field of mass spectrometry (MS) with…

② After centuries of progress, modern chemistry, now consisting of its many subdisciplines…

③ Over the past decade, microfluidics-based point-of-care (POC) diagnostics have been developed...

④ The past decade has seen the rapid development of X in many ...

5.2.3.2 总结其他的研究成果——提供背景、关键术语、概念

（1）相关文献的一般描述

① The plaques and tangles of Alzheimer's disease (AD) were first described more than a century ago.

② Here we compile and review the literature on molecular interactions as it pertains to…

（2）解释关键词

① As defined by one of its early visionaries, Prof. R. Graham Cooks, ambient ionization refers to...

② In this cornerstone masterpiece, Boyle, armed with plenty of experimental scientific methods, coined the term "analysis" describing the process of detecting the ingredients of a complex entity ...

③ Recent years have seen the development of a broad class of electrochemical biosensors, which we have termed "E-DNA sensors," that employ redox-tagged, electrode bound probe oligonucleotides.

（3）一般话题的陈述

① It is reactive toward both proteins and DNA, and forms inter-molecular cross-links between macromolecules...

② These drugs are predominantly multitargeted receptor tyrosine kinase (RTK) inhibitors approved for the treatment of cancer…

③ For small-molecule drugs, which comprise most of today's medicines...

（4）引入关键因素

① Comparing with the 14-membered erythromycin-based macrolides, 16-memberdmacrolides presents better gastrointestinal tolerance...

② The overproduction of reactive oxygen species (ROS) causes a decrease in pH and further augments oxidative stress...

③ The ability to block apoptotic signaling is a key hallmark of cancer and is thus important for oncogenesis...

5.2.3.3 引用参考文献

主语可以是研究者也可以是研究本身，取决于想强调哪个。

① This review primarily covers the most recent advancements and applications of ambient ionization MS, with a defined focus on research described in manuscripts published within the past 2 years (January 2016–September 2018).

② In 2013, Cohen and Alessi outlined some of the most important challenges that remained in kinase inhibitor drug discovery…

③ Previous methods for quantitation of PS 80 using reverse-phase (RP)-HPLC with UV detection in pharmaceutical suspension and RP-HPLC with charge aerosol detection (CAD) in protein solutions showed longer time of analysis.

5.2.3.4 问题、争议和知识缺口

① However, direct evidence to support this mechanism is sparse.

② However, the majority of kinases have been historically understudied, indicating that the field of kinase inhibitor discovery is still immature.

③ Current affinity-based target identification techniques are limited by the necessity to modify each drug individually (without losing bioactivity) ...

④ Identification and quantitative analysis of residual PS 80 often poses a challenge for...

⑤ Furthermore, leucomycin and josamycin are unstable in a low pH environment.

⑥ These newer techniques, however, are associated with their own challenges...

⑦ It is notable that a considerable part of the listed challenges is intimately related to…

⑧ However, in practice, several problems are usually encountered...

⑨ At the present, no effective therapy is available for SMA, besides supportive care.

5.2.3.5 提出你的解决方案

（1）表述本研究的目的

① This review aims to provide... / This review primarily covers...

② Here we conduct an unbiased mass-spectrometric search for...

③ In the current study, we compared the selectivity of....

④ In this study, a HPLC-CAD method was developed and validated for...

⑤ In this work, we created a single ratiometric biosensor for....

⑥ In this paper, we report an optimization strategy that....

（2）说明为什么要使用这个方法

① Here, we present a significant improvement to the PROTAC technology...

② The best method to adopt for this investigation is to...

③ A case study approach allows ...

④ The shRNA is one of the more practical ways to ...

5.2.3.6　描述过去的研究

（1）使用简单的过去时态的与时间相关的短语

① For many decades, / Since its inception in 2004, / The early 2000s brought a new age.

② Until recently, / Between 2005 and 2015, / From 2010 to 2015, / In 2020, Cohen and Alessi outlined some of the most important challenges.

（2）引用过去发表的单个的研究或者论文

① As defined by one of its early visionaries, Prof. R. Graham Cooks…

② Ambient ionization MS was first described in the literature in October of 2004...

③ BCL-2, the first identified apoptotic regulator...

（3）现在完成时用于描述最近的研究或学术活动——通常是多个研究

① Since its inception in 2004, many researchers and laboratories have contributed with approaches for...

② In the last 15 years, innovations in the field of ambient ionization MS have grown expansively.

③ As the field has grown to include many methodologies...

④ More recently, we and others have developed platform technologies...

⑤ In recent years, the field has benefited from a greater understanding of...

⑥ To date, inhibitor-induced degradation events have been discovered serendipitously rather than designed de novo.

⑦ So far, published small molecules that bind Ras have not shown this nucleotide preference.

⑧ These site-selective protein conjugation reactions have enabled the generation of protein-based probes...

⑨ Chemists have correspondingly developed a range of chemical reactions for site-specific protein modification.

⑩ Improvements in the design and analytical performance of both methods have been continuously pursued to...

⑪ Early signs of clinical antitumor activity have been observed in lymphoid malignancies.

⑫ Alzheimer's disease (AD) has become a severe social problem.

5.3 背景介绍的时态

5.3.1 现有知识

① 当陈述或报道已存在的事实时用一般现在时。

例5-4：Nature uses enzymes to install post-translational modifications onto proteins site-selectively...

② 当从很多之前的研究中报道某发现时用现在完成时。

例5-5：Previous studies have suggested the presence of an allosteric site in this region 1.

5.3.2 文献调研

① 当陈述或报道已存在的事实时用一般现在时。

例5-6：Molecular recognition in biological systems relies on the existence of specific attractive interactions between two partner molecules.

② 当引用一个单独的之前研究时用一般过去时。

例5-7：BCL-XL was subsequently identified as a related prosurvival protein and is associated with drug resistance and disease progression of multiple solid-tumor and hematological malignancies.

注意：在上面的句子中，有两个动词，was identified as 和 is associated with，第一个用过去时描述这是在过去完成的，第二个现在时是作者在现在的研究中做了什么。

③ 当从多个之前的研究中报道发现时用现在完成时。

例5-8：Previous studies showed that the abundance of NFTs correlated well with the extent of brain atrophy and cognitive decline in AD.

5.3.3 知识缺口

① 当报道已存在的事实,以及当前被接受的方法时用一般现在时。

例5-9：Spinal muscular atrophies (SMAs) are the most frequent genetic cause of infant mortality.

② 当从多个之前的研究中报道发现时，用现在完成时。

例5-10：However, liquid extraction techniques often have lower spatial resolution (600～2000 μm, with the exception of nano-DESI) than spray-based techniques (20～200 μm).

5.3.4 问题陈述

① 写和报道相关的陈述时用一般现在时。

例5-11：Here we report a photo-controlled approach to site-selective protein modification and functionalization with amine reagents.

② 写和自己的研究报道相关的陈述时用过去时。

例5-12：Upon light activation, QM was generated in proteins in situ enabling site-specific conjugation of proteins with various amine reagents as well as thiol probes.

5.3.5　其他

① 当要表达期望的结果或者提供未来的建议，用含有情态动词的一般现在时（could，may，might）。

例 5-13：We demonstrate that the QM-based Michael addition could be extended on proteins in fully aqueous and biocompatible conditions.

② 在对本研究的重要性和对未来的研究进行展望的时候，用情态动词可以使语境比较柔和。在没有确切实验证据或者研究成果未得到公认之前，切记避免使用过强或者过于肯定的语气，引起读者和审稿人的反感。

例 5-14：Using the ion funnel, an increase in the ion signal intensity from three organic acid compounds were observed, suggesting that this method could be used to improve DART detection limits.

比如上面这个例子，先引出之前观察到的一个现象，再使用情态动词表明本研究的内容。让读者在有事实依据的基础上，更容易接受你的猜测。

例 5-15：Our study further demonstrates that the Cas9 endonuclease family can be programmed with single RNA molecules to cleave specific DNA sites, thereby raising the exciting possibility of developing a simple and versatile RNA-directed system to generate dsDNA breaks (DSBs) for genome targeting and editing。

比如，Jennifer Doudna 和 Emmanuelle Charpentie 因其利用 CRISPR-Cas9 进行基因编辑的开创性研究获得 2020 年诺贝尔化学奖。奠定其学术贡献的研究工作于 2012 年发表于 Science 杂志。虽然该论文完全没有涉及基因编辑的研究，但作者在 Introduction 部分的最后一句，用 raising the exciting possibility 的句式，提出了利用 Cas9 作为基因编辑工具的可能。这样的句式既没有夸大事实，也能让人信服是他们首先提出了 CRISPR-Cas9 进行基因编辑的概念，让他们获得了在该领域内的开拓者的学术地位。

③ 引用和引语。引用（Citation）指的是用自己的话把其他作者表达的意思告诉读者。引语（Quotation）指的是直接把作者的描述原封不动的

搬过来，引语要加引号。

例 5-16：In this cornerstone masterpiece, Boyle, armed with plenty of experimental scientific methods, coined the term "analysis" describing the process of detecting the ingredients of a complex entity.

在这个例子中，"analysis"是 Boyle 创造的词汇，他是第一个使用该词汇的人，所以要加引号。

课后练习与讨论

1. 背景介绍中的六大要素是哪些？并选择几篇文献进行适当的分析。
2. 在撰写背景介绍与文献调研时会用到哪些时态？
3. 根据文献调研写作中的常用句型，练习写作技巧。
4. 选择感兴趣的一个药学研究方向或课题，检索并筛选出十篇代表性的研究性论文，尝试撰写该研究领域的背景介绍。

第 6 章 ●○

实验结果与数据处理

6.1　实验结果的写作

实验结果（Results）是指研究者通过实验操作、观测或调查所得到的结果、数据以及图像等各种资料。作为论文的核心部分，实验结果是支持科学假设、观点和结论的基础，是整个研究的价值所在。从药学专业论文写作的角度来看，首先要确定哪些实验结果是具有代表性的，并将它们按一定的逻辑顺序组织起来；其次是通过这些实验结果，验证或说明论文开始时所设定的研究目标、科学假设以及提供问题的可能答案。因此，关于实验结果的表述在论文中必须客观真实、简明扼要、准确无误，其关键点在于简单而清晰地报告实验结果。

6.1.1　实验结果的写作准备

在开始实验结果的写作之前，作者首先应该理清以下几个问题：

① 重要的发现是什么？

② 这些发现是否与期望的一致？

③ 还有哪些是可能发现却未被发现的？

在研究或调查过程中会产生大量的实验结果，既包括支持原定假设的结果，也包括不支持原定假设的结果，此外还可能得到无关或无意义的结果。论文中所呈现的实验结果应与研究主题密切相关，并具有代表性，以逻辑顺序通过表格、图形或图片的形式予以呈现；应当在开始写作之前，把图表按照最符合读者逻辑的顺序排列好；它必须能够支持引言中所陈述的最初目标或假设。然后将关键性的结果或发现与每一个数据联系起来，对这些数据逐一进行解释，排除任何与支持研究假设无关的结果，并在文本中加以必要的注释和阐述，从而对上述的问题进行回答。

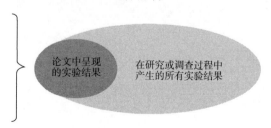

论文中所呈现的实验结果：
- ➤ 突出那些回答研究问题的实验结果（包括来自对照组的结果）
- ➤ 包含次要的实验结果
- ➤ 提供支持的信息
- ➤ 提及不支持原定假设的实验结果（与之前假设相矛盾的重要负面结果），并解释它们为什么是反常的

论文中呈现的实验结果

在研究或调查过程中产生的所有实验结果

6.1.2 实验结果的写作方法和技巧

实验结果部分的写作通常包括介绍实验结果、叙述和评论说明实验结果。

6.1.2.1 介绍实验结果

在整个实验结果部分的起始处，或者实验结果的各段落前面，给出调查实验的大致总体情况。可以使用一般现在时、现在完成时和一般过去时等多种时态来描述其他作者的工作，而仅使用一般过去时来描述自己的工作。现在完成时不用于描述自己完成的工作。关于语态，可在主动和被动语态之间切换，并取决于句子强调内容及主语部分的长度。当结果内容为主语，使用被动语态；当图表、图表名称为主语时，使用主动语态。

介绍实验结果有两种典型方法。

① 在结果部分开始，以及结果部分各段落的前面（也可在段落中），以一个句子指出反映完整研究结果的图表，**给出调查实验的大致情况，不需重复方法部分的细节**。

常用词：show, present, display, summarize, illustrate.

例6-1：Overall, the results presented below show that…

② 直接陈述结果，并在句子中插入附注，显示相关图表。

例6-2：Data in table 1 show that acupuncture technology has the potential to lower BP.

例6-3：Table 2 lists the pharmacokinetic profile in dogs of a representative set of the most optimized C-3 substituted compounds.

例6-4：Indeed, proteolysis of mTOR by thermolysin was decreased by E4 in a dose-dependent manner (Fig. 3).

例6-5：This patient experienced an exacerbation of major pre-existing CLL-related thrombocytopenia that recovered to baseline when the disseminated intravascular coagulation resolved (Fig. 4) and did not recur with subsequent longer-term re-exposure to drug (Supplementary Fig. 5).

6.1.2.2 叙述实验结果

（1）必须叙述的研究结果

① 某个参数或变量在某段时间内的变化情况。

例6-6：Blood pressure of rabbit decreased after compound A was administrated.

② 不同试样、方法或研究对象之间的比较。

例6-7：Blood pressure of rabbit decreased much lower when compared to positive agent.

③ 不同参数或变量之间的关系或影响。

例6-8：Decline of blood pressure of rabbit was related to the dosage of compound A.

在叙述研究结果时，作者需要为读者解释自己的研究结果。一般以文字叙述的方式直接告诉读者这些数据呈现何种趋势、有什么意义，并清楚地陈述根据图表中的资料所能得出的推论和结论，以及说明这些资料如何能支持自己的推论。因此，在结果部分有必要对研究结果提供一些基本的解释，以便读者能清楚、轻易地了解研究的结果。此外，如果作者觉得有必要说明自己的数据分析方法，那么在结果部分也可以作这些说明。如果研究论文有独立的讨论部分，那么对于研究结果的详细讨论应该留给讨论部分。

（2）使用时态

由于实验结果是在论文写作之前发现的，因此，它们与过去发生的事件有关，采用一般过去时。但在叙述普遍结果和理论时，采用一般现在时。

例6-9：Notably, vascular dilation and enhanced leakiness **are** hallmarks of an inflammatory stress 30. Plasma proteome analysis of CDH5-MAPK mice **demonstrated** significantly increased levels of inflammatory mediators.

例6-10：Cellular expression of bcr-abl **is** known to render myeloid cell lines growth factor independent for proliferation. The growth properties of factor-independent cell lines **were assayed** in the presence or absence of growth factor. This **is** consistent with our observation.

例6-11：To design potent small-molecule PROTACs, we **replaced** the HIF1a peptide used in previous generations of PROTAC molecules with a recently developed, high-affinity, small-molecule ligand for VHL, which **retains** the hydroxyproline moiety critical for VHL binding.

例6-12：In sharp contrast, ABT-199 **induced** a much greater immediate antileukemic effect than that previously observed with single doses of navitoclax, consistent with preclinical predictions.

例6-13：Using this approach, copper, zinc, aluminum, and nickel metal-EDTA complexes **were detected** from coins from multiple countries, including the United States, Canada, Japan, etc.

在描述实验结果时，一般建议采用客观的表述形式。

例6-14：We found that the sensitivity of the V-Chip is not as good as that of highly sophisticated clinical instruments and that the V-Chip performs better at concentrations higher than 5 ng/mL.

例6-15：It should be noted that the sensitivity of the V-Chip is not as good as that of highly sophisticated clinical instruments and that the V-Chip performs better at concentrations higher than 5 ng/mL.

例6-14与例6-15两者均可，但后者更佳。

例6-16：On the basis of its superior potency and ability to produce higher intracellular triphosphate levels, diastereomer 51 was selected as the preferred diastereomer for further study.

（3）向读者说明数据的价值比仅仅展示它们更重要

例6-17：The LOD and LOQ of PS 80 was found to be more detectable with GC-MS than the HPLC-ELSD technique.

例6-18：The LOD and LOQ of PS 80 was found to be 0.30g/mL and 0.91g/mL respectively over the range of 0.5～100g/mL using GC-MS and 2.80g/mL and 8.48g/mL respectively over the range of 5.0～750g/mL using HPLC-ELSD method. The GC-MS technique was observed to be more sensitive than HPLC-ELSD.

在例6-17中，形容词 "detectable" 对作者来说是非常明确且容易理解，但对于那些没有办法理解在论文中为什么 "GC-MS more detectable" 的读者来说，这样的描述性形容词 (interesting, sensitive, suitable) 并没有传递出任何有科学依据的内容。需要给读者足够的信息，让他们能够从结果中自然地得出"more detectable"的结论，即告诉读者为什么"more detectable"。例6-18通过突出强调 GC-MS 与 HPLC-ELSD 数据的对比来告诉读者为什么"more detectable"。

（4）精确描述图表中所展示的数据或结果

例6-19：Supplementary Fig.7 shows the relationship between cellular toxicity and concentrations.

例6-20：No cellular toxicity was observed at any concentration（Supplementary Fig.7）.

在例6-19中，作者只是告诉读者能够从图中看到哪些信息。但例6-20则更侧重于向读者展示从图中数据可推理出的结论。例6-19迫使读者根据数据自行得出结论，而且不一定是正确的结论。而例6-19则减少了读者不必要的思考，让读者正确理解数据中传达的结论。同时还需注意，避免使用"can be seen"和"we can see"这样的短语，建议将图或表引用放在句尾的括号中。

如果结果与讨论这两个部分是分开写的，那么在结果部分则不需要过分地解释或分析数据，留待讨论部分加以说明。

例6-21：The duration of exposure to running water had a pronounced effect on cumulative seed germination percentages (Fig. 2). Seeds exposed to the 2days treatment had the highest cumulative germination (84%), 1.25 times that of the 12h or 5days group sand four times that of controls.

例6-22：The results of the germination experiment (Fig. 2) suggest that the optimal time for running-water treatment is 2 days. This group showed the highest cumulative germination (84%), with longer (5 d) or shorter (12 h) exposures producing smaller gains in germination when compared to the control group.

在例6-21中，作者强调了他们希望读者关注的趋势或差异，并没有给出主观的解释。而在例6-22中，将观察到的结果分析后得到最优条件的结论。如果结果与讨论部分分开，则例6-21的写作方式合适。如果结果与讨论合二为一，则例6-22的写作方式更为合适。

6.1.2.3 评论或说明实验结果

介绍一个或一系列实验结果后，加以评论说明；再介绍另一个或一系列实验结果，加以评论说明。这种类型在段落末尾或整个实验结果部分的结尾处较多见，时态可采用一般现在时或一般过去时。

① 根据本人的研究结果作出推论。常用句型如 The results suggest that...

② 作者解释研究结果或说明产生研究结果的原因。常用句型如 These findings are understandable because...

③ 作者对此次研究结果与其他研究者曾发生的结果作比较。常用句型如 These results agree with Garner's analysis, in that...

④ 作者对自己的研究方法或技术的性能与其他研究者的方法技术的性能进行比较。例如 The recognition rate of our system is significantly higher than that reported for Token's system.

或者采取介绍数个研究结果后，对所有结果作出精简的说明或评论。请参考例 6-23～例 6-25。

例6-23：Taken together, these data demonstrated that chronic activation of endothelial MAPK adversely impacts steady-state hematopoiesis and HSC function.

例6-24：Collectively, these findings suggested that increased NF-κB signaling within ECs of CDH5-MAPK mice drives an inflammatory stress response leading to vascular defects.

例6-25：The results showed that the RSDs were 4.06%, 1.66% and 0.71% at the concentration of 5 g/mL, 50 g/mL and 100 g/mL, respectively. The RSDs were 9.72%, 6.84% and 3.44% for inter-day precision, respectively.

当对结果提出可能解释和说明时，并以研究结果为据作出推论时，句子常用 appear、suggest、seem 等推测动词或情态动词 may。如果对实验结果的说明具有普遍有效性，通常使用一般现在时。如果在评论内容中比较作者与其他文献的研究结果时，由于这种比较是不受时间影响的逻辑关系，因此可以用一般现在时；但如果作者认为实验结果说明只限定在本人的特定研究条件中，则使用一般过去时。请参考例 6-26 和例 6-27。

例6-26：It seems that this period takes generally 3 or 4 weeks for COVID-19.

例6-27：These data are the first demonstration of a high affinity PPAR ligand and provide strong evidence that PPARγ is a molecular target for the adipogenic effects of thiazolidinediones.

6.1.3　实验结果部分的写作质量评估

当完成实验结果部分的写作时，认真核对以下问题，以评估该部分的写作质量，是否简单而清晰地报告了实验结果：

① 是否选择了代表性的实验结果，以回答在前言部分设置的问题以及基于此所得到的可靠结论？

② 是否已经尽可能清楚地表达了研究者的想法，能够为审稿人和读者充分理解本研究结果带来明显的帮助？

③ 是否选择了最好的方式来展示实验数据和结果（如图形、图片或表格）？是否确保这些图形、图片和表格中的数据之间没有重复或遗漏？

④ 是否已经准确地报告了论文中每个图和表所传达的关键结果或趋势，而不是简单地向审稿人和读者重复图表中的数据？

⑤ 是否客观地描述了图表和数据，而非过分解释且基于此得出不可靠的结论？

⑥ 是否提到了论文中所采用的实验方法可能会影响到的实验结果？

⑦ 是否正确地使用了时态和语态？一般过去时表示自己的发现（常用被动形式），一般现在时表示对已确立的科学事实的描述（被动和主动语态均可）。

6.1.4　实验结果的写作范例

例6-28：药物分子的合成路线（*J. Med. Chem.* **2014**, 57, 2033.；已获授权许可，版权所有©2014 美国化学会）：写作上采用时间的逻辑先后顺序，从起始原料或关键中间体出发得到最终产物，应体现出关键反应以及重要的反应试剂等。

In a novel process, fluorene **39a** could be difluorinated by treatment with KHMDS in the presence of *N*-fluorobenzene sulfonimide (Scheme 16) to give **39b**. The iodine-bearing carbon of **39b** was selectively metalated by reaction with *i*-

PrMgCl and converted to single chloroketone **39c** by quenching the Grignard species with the Weinreb amide 2-chloro-*N*-methoxy-*N*-methylacetamide. Carboxylic acid **12** was alkylated with **39c**, and the resulting ketoester was condensed to imidazole **39d** by heating with ammonium acetate. **39d** was coupled to **38a**, providing **39e**. Boc-removal was followed by peptide coupling with **11** to afford **39**.

(a)*N*-Fluorobenzenesulfonimide, KHMDS, THF; (b) *i*-PrMgCl, 2-chloro-*N*-methoxy-*N*-methylacetamide, THF; (c) **12**, K₂CO₃, KI, acetone; (d) NH₄OAc, PhMe; (e) **38a**, Pd(OAc)₂, PPh₃, NaHCO₃, DME/H₂O; (f) HCl/dioxane/DCM; (g) **11**,HATU, *i*-Pr₂NEt, DMF

例6-29：小分子-蛋白质的共晶结构及作用方式（*J. Med. Chem.* **2017**，60，8369.；经授权许可，版权所有©2017，美国化学会）：根据小分子与蛋白质结合的重要性，依次阐述其作用力。并可进一步探讨结合口袋的特点，指出哪些作用力可能更为关键，是否有新的结合模式指导后续药物分子的设计。

An X-ray cocrystal structure of sulfonamide **24** (PDB code: 5UVX) in BRD4 BDⅡ (Figure 4) confirmed the presence of a productive hydrogen bond between the NH of Asp381 and one of the sulfonamide oxygens, with a measured distance of 2.8Å. Notably, the positioning of the sulfonamide moiety allowed for the formation of this hydrogen bond without disturbing the valuable interactions between the pyrrolopyridone carbonyl (2.9 Å) and the pyrrole NH (2.9 Å) with Asn433 and also maintained the critical position of the phenyl ether in the WPF pocket.

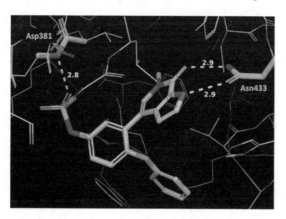

Figure 4. Compound **24** (yellow) bound to BRD4 BDⅡ （resolution=1.5Å，PDB code 5UVX）. Leu385 removed for clarity.

例6-30：化合物系列的构效关系（SAR）（*J. Med. Chem.* **2014**，57，2033.；经授权许可，版权所有©2014，美国化学会）：需要突出化学结构/基团的改变对生物活性的影响，是增加了还是降低了，改变的幅度多大？通过系列的构效关系研究，发现最优的药物分子。

Cmpd	X	EC$_{50}$（GT1a）/ (nmol/L)	EC$_{50}$（GT1b）/ (nmol/L)
16	bond	>44	35
17		>44	0.14
18		11	0.026
19		1.7	0.01
20		0.11	0.004
21		0.20	0.016
22		0.50	0.009
23		3.7	0.044

A value of >44 nmol/L means that no inhibition was observed at this top well concentration.

Directly linked bis-benzimidazole **16** and monoalkyne inhibitor **17** showed no inhibitory activity under the assay conditions (up to 44 nmol/L), whereas diyne **18** had an EC$_{50}$ of 11 nmol/L. Replacing the alkynes with a thiophene ring (**19**) improved potency 6-fold, and the benzimidazole-phenyl-benzimidazole core in **22** provided further improvements in potency (EC$_{50}$=500 pmol/L). Replacement of phenyl with biphenyl decreased activity 7-fold. Finally, insertion of fused ring systems provided highly potent naphthyl inhibitor **20**(EC$_{50}$=109 pmol/L), with benzodithiophene **21** only 2-fold less active. From these studies, inhibitors with fused central ring systems, as in **20** and **21**, were the most potent, whereas less lipophilic connectors, such as in alkynes **17** or **18**, afforded weaker activity.

例6-31：化合物的体内药理药效学结果（*J. Med. Chem.* **2017**，60，8369.；经授权许可，版权所有©2017. 美国化学会）：化合物本身的抗肿瘤效果如何？与阳性药比，有何突出优势？是否具有毒性或其他问题？

In vivo antitumor efficacy of compound **63** is exemplified by activity in a Kasumi-1 AML mouse xenograft model shown in Figure 7. Compound **63** was dosed orally QD at 1 mg/kg for 25 days and achieved 99% tumor growth inhibition (TGI) with acceptable tolerability (weight loss≤10%). For comparison a representative therapy for AML, 5-azacitidine, achieved 76% TGI when administered at its MTD (IV Q7d, 8 mg/kg).

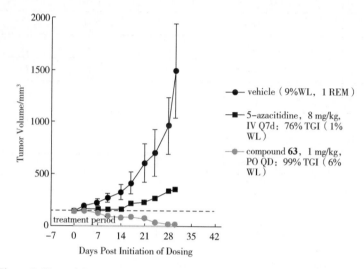

Figure 7. Kasumi-1 mouse xenograft study with compound **63**. Values represent mean±SE（*n*=8/group）；WL=maximum mean weight loss；REM=removed from study due to morbidity.

例6-32：Characterization of stem cell and transient amplifying cell populations from DU145 cells.（*Sci. Rep.* **2020**, 10, 70948.）

We first determined the characteristics of stem and non-stem cell populations in DU145 cells, based on the expression of stem (CD133), basal (CD44) and luminal (CD24) cell surface markers. Flow cytometry analysis showed that CSCs (CD133+/CD44+) were detected as a small population in DU145 cells (1044%), while the most abundant population (85.74%) was represented by TA/CB cells (CD44+/CD24+) (Fig.1a). **We then sorted** CSCs and TA/CB populations based on the expression of the same surface markers and sought to determine their characteristics. Sorted CSCs showed higher expression levels of the stemness genes CD133, CD44 and ALDH1A1, compared to TA/CB cells (Fig.1b). **Furthermore, we found** that cells from both populations were able to form colonies (Fig.1c) and spheres (Fig.1d) when grown in vitro. **Notably,** spheres derived from CSCs (CD133+/CD44+) showed higher expression of CD133, CD44 and ALDH1A1 (Fig.1e) as well as higher levels of the STAT3-target genes c-myc, Bcl-xl, Mcl-1 and Survivin compared to spheres derived from TA/CB cells (CD44+/CD24+) (Fig.1f). **Furthermore,** immunocytochemistry analysis on sorted cells from DU145 showed that CSCs express higher levels of active phosphorylated STAT3 (pSTAT3) compared to the TA/CB population (Fig.1g). **Altogether**, **these data indicate** that CD133$^+$/CD44$^+$ cells and their derived spheres retain stemness characteristics and show high activity of STAT3, in agreement with previously published work.

6.1.5　实验结果的常用表达句型

（1）检查/调查

例6-33：Precision-cut lung slice (PCLS) is a novel versatile tool to **examine** host-pathogen interaction in the chicken lung.

例6-34：Drug development for AD therapies can be examined by **inspecting** the drug development pipeline as represented on clinicaltrials.

（2）治疗

例6-35：Several miRNA-targeted therapeutics have reached clinical deve-lopment, including antimiRs targeted at miR-122, which reached phage Ⅱ trials for **treating** hepatitis.

例6-36：The diagnosis is made through doppler ultrasonography, but the best **therapeutical** option is still matter of debate.

（3）用药

例6-37：In the prevention study, HK-2 was **administered** orally beginning 5 days before the start of the noise and ending 10 days after the noise.

例6-38：STS **in combination with** PD-1 blockade has a therapeutic effect against lung cancer.

（4）作用

例6-39：**Effects** of fermented milk, citrulline and Lactobacillus helveticus ASCC 511 on IPEC-J2 cell growth.

例6-40：When cells are exposed to electric fields, electrical stresses **act on** their surfaces.

（5）比较

例6-41：We also observed **common** variant enrichment in two developmental pathways that can be pharmacologically modulated.

例6-42：The pair-level physiological **similarity** was also higher compared to the shielded condition.

例6-43：Fecal luminal bacterial composition **differs** between IBS patients and healthy subjects.

（6）目的

例6-44：The **aim** of this study is to establish a mathematical model for managing sunitinib-induced hypertension and blood pressure fluctuation.

例6-45：This study tested a framework in which **goals** are proposed to be central determinants of achievement patterns.

（7）程度

例6-46：We found a net increase in the **extent** of neutral lipids including saturated and monounsaturated FA in response to TGF-β2 stimulation for 6 h.

例6-47：Compared with the wild type HBx, mutants MT2-3 and MT20-21 had a significantly lower **degree** of association with cccDNA.

（8）原因

例6-48：Exogenous expression of C-terminal DISC1 mutant **causes** loss of dendritic spines and aggregates within dendrites.

例6-49：The remaining variants were downgraded **due to** the lack of similar evidence.

（9）变化

例6-50：Progressive **decline** in lung function is the hallmark of chronic obstructive pulmonary disease.

例6-51：The polymorphism in the human μ-opioid receptor gene may **increase** morphine requirements in patients with pain caused by malignant disease.

（10）表明/说明

例6-52：Our findings **demonstrate** that chronic endothelial inflammation adversely impacts niche activity and HSC function which is reversible upon suppression of inflammation.

例6-53：Figure 11 **illustrates** how mutations in a group of four samples can be compressed into four bits.

6.2 数据及图像处理要求

科研论文需要真实可靠的实验数据支撑所提出的科学假说，是科研论文的核心部分。在撰写论文前需对所有已获得的实验数据进行整理和汇总，选定最具代表性的结果，即选择能够支持或回答论文的目标、假说或科学问题的结果，并将其按一定的逻辑顺序排列。对原始数据及图像的处理是该过程中的重要步骤，正确的处理方法和恰当的数据展示形式能够快速吸引读者的注意，与文字描述相结合，使读者正确理解论文的思路。

6.2.1 数据处理的目的和基本原则

① 数据处理的首要目的是通过对数据的归纳和整合，帮助读者快速并正确理解论文的设计思路，阐明论文提出科学问题的合理性或支持所提出假说的正确性。

② 将数据以图表的形式展示可简洁有效地列举大量精确数据或资料，直观、有效地展现复杂数据间的比较、关联、趋势等。

③ 根据所选期刊对图表数量的要求，选择最具代表性的、可直接支持实验假说或验证实验结果的核心数据，置于科研论文的正文部分，其余次要数据可排列于补充材料（Supporting Information）中。每个数据的选择都要有明确的目的性和必要性，在此基础上，对数据的处理及其呈现形式的选择很重要。

④ 数据的呈现形式应简洁明了，使读者易于理解。对于由多幅数据图表组成的组图，各图间的排列顺序同样应遵循论文的写作逻辑进行排列，使读者在阅读文字的同时，能够快速定位对应的数据，正确解读实验结果。

⑤ 论文中的每个图表（包括补充材料）都需附有清晰的图题、图注。

⑥ 文字与图表的内容应避免重复。对于简单的数据，可用文本说明的，

无须再以图表形式展示。对于复杂或重要的核心数据，需采用图表的形式呈现，对应文字部分应是对数据的进一步解析，而非简单的重复描述数据内容。

⑦ 相同数据采用文字或不同的图表形式展示会产生不同的视觉效果，因此在整理数据阶段，应充分考虑并选择合适的数据展示形式。

比如，在对液相洗脱条件进行描述时，可采用文字直接描述的形式"A gradient elution condition was applied as follows: 0% B for 0~5 min, 0%~6% B for 5~20min, and 6%~40% B for 20~50 min; 40%~0% B for 50~51 min, and re-equilibrated for 51~65 min." 也可采用如下例子中所示的表格或折线图予以展示。文字描述虽可提供液相洗脱条件的准确信息，但相比而言，以表格或折线图形式展示则更为简洁明了，使读者能直观观察到流动相比例的变化趋势。

例6-54：同一数据的不同展示形式（*J. Pharm. Biomed. Anal.* **2010**, 51, 24.；已获授权许可）

（1）表格形式展示数据

Table. Gradient program proposed for the analysis of OT and its related substrates.

Time/min	Mobile Phase A（*V/V*）/%	Mobile Phase B（*V/V*）/%	Notes
0~5	100	0	Isocratic
5~20	100~94	0~6	Linear gradient
20~50	94~60	6~40	Linear gradient
50~51	60~100	40~0	Linear gradient
51~65	100	0	Isocratic reequlibration

（2）折线图形式展示数据

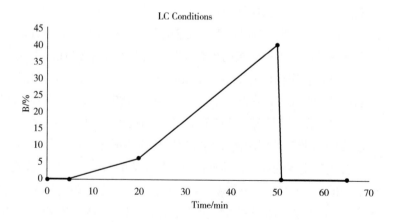

6.2.2　图表的准备

① 数据处理及图表绘制均应采用专业软件进行（如 Adobe Illustrator、GraphPad、Word 或 Excel 等），操作方便的同时不会降低数据图像原有的清晰度和分辨率。

② 图表中文字需统一，包括字体和字号等，同时需符合期刊的要求。

③ 单个图表中所包含的信息应完整。若一个结论由多个数据共同支持，可将相关数据以组图形式展示，在建立组图时，应充分考虑各数据图表间关联。相反，不宜将具有多个不同的结论或重点的数据图表组合成一个整体，以组图的形式展示，避免给读者的阅读和理解造成困难。

④ 对于包含多个数据图表的组图，各数据图表通常以英文字母（A～Z）标明顺序，且排列顺序应与论文的写作逻辑相符，不同刊物对大小写及特定字体有具体要求，在作图时需充分考虑。

⑤ 图表在论文中的排布需充分考虑美观和协调，不应在一完整段落中插入图表。

⑥ 按各期刊正式发表时的要求，调整图表的比例，如单栏或双栏，长宽的尺寸要求等；在调整的同时需保证不降低图表的清晰度和分辨率。

⑦ 需合理控制图表的长度，应尽量避免在正式发表时出现跨页的情况。

⑧ 对于需要读者在阅读时进行对比的数据，所用的标准（如单位、横纵坐标范围、标尺、缩写等）应保持一致。

⑨ 图表不必做得过于花哨（如增加不必要的三维立体、阴影或边框等效果）。

⑩ 对于极少数阴性对照或确无展示必要的数据，可用"data not shown"叙述。

6.2.3　表格（Table）

表格用于展示实验过程中获得的具有确切数值的数据信息；或数据量较大时，常用表格形式总结，如定量数据、分子量、回收率、检测强度或组学相关数据等。

① 表格的设计应合理且符合逻辑，遵循一定的实验记录过程或运算顺序，有利于读者阅读和分析。如例 6-55 中需向读者展示实验过程中检测

到重要肽段相关信息时，首先列出所检测的肽段序列，其次列出每一肽段对应的理论质荷比和实验测得的质荷比，最后对比两者之间的差异，通过计算得到置信度，即 confidence，符合思考及计算的逻辑。

② 表格由行和列组成，应清楚写出对应的行标题和列标题，通常以单词或短语形式描述其所对应数值的含义。

③ 表格中包含的各数值或变量的单位应统一列于行或列标题中，包括%，避免写于各数值后，重复赘述，如例 6-56。

④ 同一类型数据的表现形式应一致，如例 6-56，包括保留小数位数、有效数字等。表中同一列下的数据保留小数位数均相同，不同列之间根据实际需要可有所区别。

⑤ 避免出现空白单元格，如确无数据的单元格，应以 N/A 等表示。

⑥ 建议使用三线表形式展示数据。

⑦ 需要特别说明的内容可以脚注的方式加以说明,如数据处理过程中所采用的计算公式、数学模型或在表格中出现的缩略语等。

此外，表格也常出现在综述文章中，便于总结凝练信息，如对比不同方法的优缺点、展现某种技术发展历史中的重要时间节点，或总结归纳重要文献以便于索引，使读者一目了然。如例 6-57 所示，表格用于总结及对比常用的化学蛋白质组学方法的优缺点。将大量信息进行汇总，使读者一目了然。

例 6-55：表格的设计及数据展示的逻辑（*J. Med. Chem.* **2020**，63，816.；已获授权许可，版权所有©2020 美国化学会）

Tabel. Peptide mass fingerprinting for recombinant chymase.

Fragment Sequence	Theoretical [M+H]$^+$	Observed [M+H]$^+$	Confidence
MAYL EIVTSNGPSKF	1672.80	1672.69	99%
NFVLTAAHCAGR	1224.64	1224.55	99%
QKL EVIK	839.51	839.45	99%
VAGWGR	676.33	676.28	99%
ISHYRPWINQIL QAN	1852.96	1852.83	99%

例 6-56：表格中数据格式统一（*J. Pharm. Biomed. Anal.* **2019**，174，161.；已获授权许可）

Table. Within-day accuracy and precision and between-day accuracy and precision results of the assay.

Matrix	Sample	Within-day[a] accuracy/%	Between-day[a] accuracy/%	Within-day[b] precision/%	Between-day[b] precision/%
Plasma	LLOQ	110.3	99.9	6.7	9.3
	QC-L	86.6	96.3	9.6	8.8
	QC-M	105.7	102.5	5.4	3.8
	QC-H	105.1	103.2	5.4	1.9
	ULOQ	113.6	106.6	5.6	5.5
Matrix	Sample	Within-day[a] accuracy/%	Between-day[a] accuracy/%	Within-day[b] precision/%	Between-day[b] precision/%
Urine	LLOQ	113.0	109.0	1.0	4.1
	QC-L	108.7	103.0	2.4	4.8
	QC-M	104.3	101.6	3.2	2.2
	QC-H	107.6	103.2	1.4	3.7
	ULOQ	108.6	104.9	2.2	2.9

a. The accuracy values represent the deviation of the measured concentrations compared to the theoretical concentrations, expressed as a percentage of the theoreticalconcentrations.

b. The precision values are expressed as coeficients of variation. All values should be within the acceptance criteria of±20% for the LLOQ samples and±15% for the otherQC samples.

例 6-57：以表格形式汇总大量信息（*Pharmacol. Therapeut.* **2016**，162，10.；已获授权许可）

Table. Comparison of quantitative proteomics approaches applied to chemical proteomics target identification that are discussed in the present review.

Strategies	Metabolic labeling (SILAC)	Chemical labeling (iTRAQ)	Label-free (Spectra counting or emPAI)
Advantages	Labeling at protein level before enrichment Labeling efficiency can be well controlled Can avoid the variation in the pull-down process (higher consistency and accuracy)	Straightforward labeling at peptide level Suitable for almost all different kinds of samples High-throughput and multiplexing (up to 8 samples can be compared in a single LC-MS run) Convenient and less time-consuming	Convenient to use Do not need isotopic labeling Cheap Simple workflow
Disadvantages	Labeling processes take long time Usually the comparison limits to 2~3 conditions Cell culture systems only Not suitable for cells that cannot be maintained for a long time (platelets or primary cells)	Variation introduced during protein digestion, pull-down, or peptide labeling	Semi-quantitative Less accurate Need to maintain consistent LC-MS running conditions
Sample types	Cultured cells which can incorporate the stable isotope-labeled amino acids	Any samples (cultured cells, tissues, body fluids, etc.)	Any samples (cultured cells, tissues, body fluids, etc.)

6.2.4　图（Figure）

图的类型众多，在药学专业论文写作中应选择最能够清楚表述数据的类型，以简明清晰为前提，避免将多个图或不同类型的图以复杂的形式组合，增加读者的阅读困难。

（1）图形（如散点图、柱状图）

散点图、柱状图等可用于展示两个或以上数据间的关系，如变化趋势或占比信息等，常用于需要读者对不同数据进行比较的情况，如趋势、占比、实验对象随实验条件变化情况等（如例6-58所示）。

① X 轴表示自变量，Y 轴表示因变量。

② 坐标轴应从零开始，选取适当的坐标范围。如果数据间的跨度很大，且在某段区间内无显著趋势变化时，则可采取坐标轴中间断开的形式，重点展示变化趋势显著的部分，使数据更加精练。如例6-59所示，横坐标中25～40间跨度较大，但无数据点，因此采取横坐标断开的方式，使数据点更加集中且美观，同时使图中数据趋势变化更加显著。

③ 坐标轴应有对应的标题，标题中应包括坐标轴对应的变量和单位，缺一不可。

④ 对于表示统计学结果的图，包含趋势线、公式等信息应标记清楚；应尽量使用通用的符号表示特定含义，如星号（*）表示具有统计学意义等。

⑤ 图中的标注应清晰，包括数字、字母等，不能因过小而被读者忽略，造成表述不清或信息的缺失。

⑥ 若图形中包含多个数据集或趋势线，需用不同颜色或不同形状图形区分，并在图内加以说明（如例6-60所示）。

例6-58：突出不同数据间的对比关系（*Talanta* **2006**，68，908.；已获授权许可）

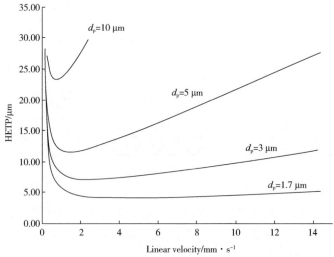

Fig.1. Van Deemter curves for different particle sizes（10 μm，5 μm，3 μm，1.7 μm）.

例6-59：以断点形式展示数据（*PLoS ONE* **2015**，10，e0115973.；已
获授权许可）

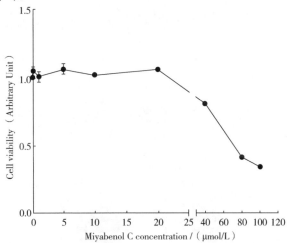

例6-60：多个数据集的展示（*J. Med. Chem.* **2019**，62，10342.；已获
授权许可，版权所有©2019美国化学会）

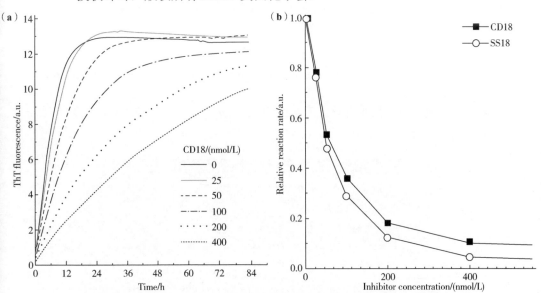

Figure s9.(a) Influence of αSyn dimer CD18 on firillization of αSyn (50 μmol/L) in the presence of
seeds (0.5 μmol/L).(b) Relative initial fibrillization rate as a function of CD18 dimer concentration,
calculated from data shown in the panel A compared with the data for SS18.

（2）示意图

示意图通常用于向读者展示实验流程、总结新颖的实验设计流程（如

例 6-61 所示）、实验过程中所使用的特定仪器或装置的说明，或其他用文本无法充分说明的信息。也常用在综述中，总结或列举方法的用途，随时间的发展历程等（如例 6-62 和例 6-63 所示）。

例6-61：实验流程图（*Chem. Biol.* **2013**，20，667.；已获授权许可）

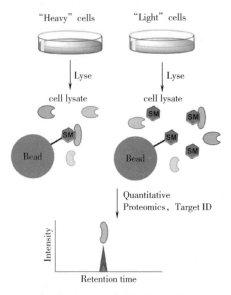

Figure 1. Affinity Capture Coupled to SILAC for Small Molecule Target Identification

例6-62：展示并总结方法的用途（*Anal. Chem.* **2015**，87，1437.；已获授权许可）

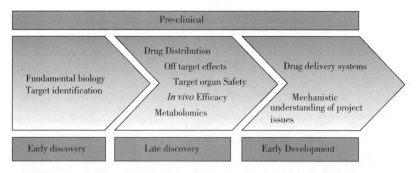

Figure 1. Overview of where MSI is able to impact preclinical drug discovery/ development.

例6-63：总结方法学发展的时间线（*Analyst* **2013**，138, 5519.；已获授权许可）

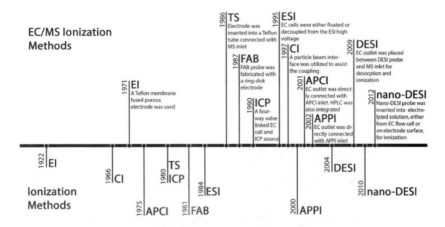

Fig.1   Timelines for the development of EC/MS and ionization methods.

（3）图片

图片是最常用的数据展示形式，可直观地展示实验结果。

① 应具备高清晰度及高分辨率，包含必要的说明，如显微或扫描电镜结果的放大倍数应以图示法（标尺刻度）表示（如例 6-64 所示）。

② 图中若有需要读者特别注意或需重点关注的数据，可采用箭头或其他具有标识性的图表指出具体位置（如例 6-65 所示）。任何出现在图表中的，非数据本身的符号、字母、数字或颜色变化等，必须在图注中或采用脚注的形式详细说明其含义。

③ 对于论文中涉及的重要化合物结构式或化学反应方程式，也可以图片形式置于正文中，帮助读者了解化合物性质或文章中所涉及的重要化学反应原理，避免使用冗长的文字描述（如例 6-66 和例 6-67 所示）。

例6-64：电镜图（*ACS Chem. Neurosci.* **2019**，10，3510.；已获授权许可，版权所有©2019 美国化学会）

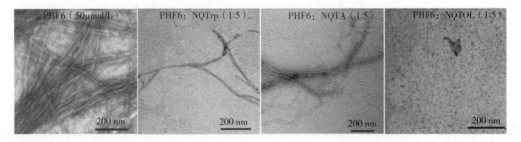

例 6-65：以箭头标注需读者特别注意之处（*PLoS One* **2013**，8，e74104.；已获授权许可）

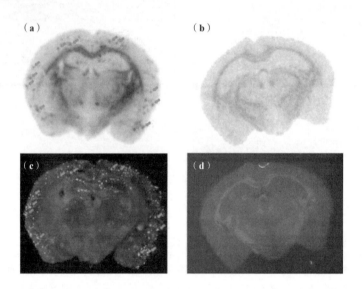

例6-66：药物分子的化学结构式

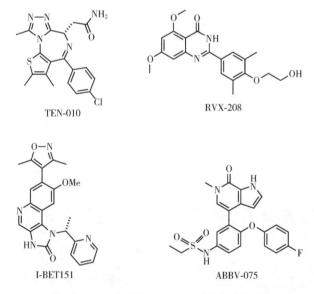

TEN-010

RVX-208

I-BET151

ABBV-075

Fig. Selective BET Inhibitors in Clinical Trials

药学专业论文写作

6.2.5　图题图例（Figure legend）的撰写原则

图题图例的撰写原则如下：

① 所有的图表都应配有相应的图例，使读者无需阅读文章具体内容的情况下也能够准确了解图表中数据所代表的含义，包括使用的方法，观察到的结果等，切忌仅简单重复描述数据。

② 图题和图例中不应描述图表中未展示的结果。

③ 图题通常可用一个单词或短语表示，图例则可以是完整的句子，但不宜过长，不宜在图例中对数据进行解析。

④ 图例中应简要说明图片内容，同时解释图中出现的数字、符号或颜色变化等特殊标注的含义；针对组图的图例，应根据组图中各小图编号顺序依次对其进行解释。

⑤ 撰写图例时应提前了解拟投期刊对于图例是否有单词数要求。

⑥ 图例表达不尽处，可加入脚注对其加以解释。

⑦ 对于图中涉及的缩写或表中运用到的计算公式等，除在正文中对其进行必要的解释外，在图例中也应有相对应的说明。

⑧ 图题图例的表述通常采用现在时。

⑨ Table 的图题写于表格上方，Figure 的图题写于图下方。

⑩ 正文中的图表以 Table 或 Figure 标记，补充材料中的图表以 Table S 或 Figure S 标记。

例6-67：正文中的图例（*Nature* **2013**，503，548.；已获授权许可）

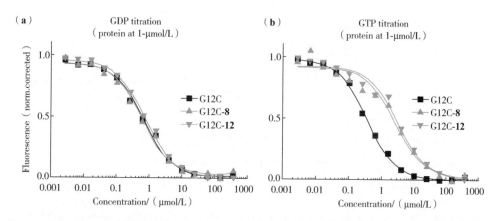

Figure 3

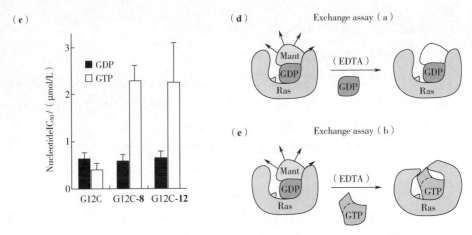

Figure 3　Compound binding to S-IIP changes nucleotide preference of K-Ras from GTP to GDP.
(**a**) EDTA-mediated competition between mant-dGDP loaded on K-Ras (G12C) and free unlabelled GDP.
The experiment was carried out with full-length K-Ras (G12C) alone (squares), or modified by **8**
(upwards triangles) or **12** (downwards triangles) (n=3). Data from a representative experiment is
shown ftted to a sigmoidal curve for each protein. (**b**) EDTA-mediated competition between
bound mant-dGDP and free unlabelled GTP. (**c**) Quantification of the GDP and GTP
titrations in a and b (n=3; error bars denote s.d; IC_{50} obtained from sigmoidal fits).
(**d**)、(**e**) Schematic representation of experiments shown in a (d) and b (e).

课后练习与讨论

1. 实验结果部分的撰写过程中有哪些注意事项？
2. 为什么论文中只是部分呈现了科研过程中的实验结果？作为作者的你该如何选取这些材料？
3. 如何确保实验结果部分的写作质量？
4. 数据处理应该遵循哪些规范？
5. 如何选择合适的图表清晰明确地呈现实验结果？
6. 图表制作中需要注意哪些事项？
7. 根据范例，尝试将实验结果的写作技巧与方法运用到自己的论文写作中。

第 7 章　●○

讨论与结论

7.1 讨论的写作

讨论（Discussion）是指对实验结果的深入解释及探讨，通过与现有知识（既包括他人发表的成果，也包括研究者自己的前期发现）的比较，分析论文所用研究方法或所得结果的优势及不足。讨论部分是桥接实验结果与结论的重要环节，也是向读者强调研究发现正确性与重要性的最佳时机，并能为相关领域提供新的研究方向、观点或者技术。

一般而言，讨论是论文中最重要但也是最难写好的部分，是论文被拒稿或质疑的重要原因。即使用母语写作，写好讨论部分也相当不易。作者写作前应对相关研究领域进行详尽的文献调研与归纳，充分掌握研究现状和存在的问题，为写好讨论部分奠定基础。写作时应仔细斟酌，将数据或问题分析清楚，并对本人研究发现有客观公正的评价。部分期刊或同一期刊的部分文章将"讨论（Discussion）"与"结果（Results）"合在一起，作为"Results and Discussion"，而非单独撰写，因此需认真研读投稿指南，同时分析目标期刊的其他作者如何撰写讨论部分，进而结合自身情况，确定并完善文章的构架。

相比背景介绍（Introduction）部分，讨论部分更依赖作者的专业知识、写作功底以及逻辑思维能力，在撰写上没有固定的套路。但一般而言，药学专业论文的讨论部分包括以下几个方面：

① 客观陈述实验结果，说明数据能否支持论文开始时的实验假说。

② 与已有文献相比，实验结果有何异同？

③ 深入探讨并诠释研究发现，对于非预期或与文献报道不同的结果，应有合理的解释。

④ 本研究有何优势？研究发现能否提高人们对此领域的认识？

⑤ 本研究有何不足？列举所有可能影响实验结果的因素。

⑥ 说明本研究的结论和意义，以及对相关领域可能产生的影响或启示。

⑦ 针对本研究尚未解决的问题或者局限，指出将来的研究方向。

7.1.1 讨论部分的开始

万事开头难，讨论部分的撰写也是如此。需要注意的是，讨论与结果不同，不能过多地罗列或重复结果部分的内容。可以采用以下多种方式开始讨论的撰写。

（1）简要介绍研究目标和内容

例7-1：In this study, we develop a delicate *ex-vivo* BBB model based on millimeter-scale engineered neural construct with well controlled vasculature network.（*Biomaterials* **2020**, 245, 119980.）

例7-2：In this study, novel dual-crosslinked MC-Tyr hydrogels were successfully synthesized via two-step reactions.（*Carbohydr. Polym.* **2020**, 238, 116192.）

例7-3：Here, we addressed this challenge by introducing a library of 12 complementary network bioinks comprising photocrosslinkable hydrogels (various forms of gelatin, hyaluronic acid, chondroitin sulfate, dextran, alginate, chitosan, heparin, and PEG) supplemented with 5 wt % gelatin.（*Sci. Adv.* **2020**, 6, eabc5529.）

（2）回顾在前言（Introduction）部分中提出的科学问题、实验假说或预测

例7-4：These previous reports led us to investigate that whether the detoxification capacity of tobacco-specific carcinogens varied between COPD smokers and control smokers, as a potential, additional risk factor for COPD development.（*Free Radic. Biol. Med.* **2021**, 164, 99.）

例7-5：Because electrophiles derived from lipid oxidation react with macromolecules such as histones or DNA, they represent ideal candidates to explain the molecular perturbations that are associated with carcinogenesis.（*Gastroenterology* **2021**, 160, 1256.）

例7-6：In our previous work, we found that anthocyanins could significantly inhibit the protein and mRNA expression of CYP2E1. Hence, the decrease of GA-VAL probably contributed to the blocking of AA epoxidation to GA by BAE.（*Food Chem.* **2019**, 274, 611.）

例7-7：This is primarily based on the hypothesis that the genotoxic PAHs, such as those studied herein, act via similar modes/mechanisms of action.（*Arch. Toxicol.* **2016**, 90, 2461.）

例7-8：What then are the possible explanations for the poor IVIVE predictability? It could be that all or some of the published measurements of CLH, *in vivo*, CLint, *in vitro*, fu, B, and QH are invalid. This could be, but since many of these parameters have been investigated by many scientists, with a reasonable degree of concordance, this is probably not the answer. Let us look now at the individual parameters. （*AAPS J.* **2020**, 22, 120.）

（3）概述研究结果中最重要的内容

例7-9：The strategy includes a predicted MRM list of 36 ion pairs based on MS fragmentation patterns of known DNA adducts, and authentic standards were synthesized to confirm the reaction sites of the unknown DNA adducts. 7PrG and 7BuG were clearly discovered and identified *in vitro* using this strategy. （*Talanta* **2021**, 222, 121500.）

例7-10：In this study, we further advanced this methodology for DPC quantification using a state-of-the-art Orbitrap MS with high mass resolution and accuracy. （*Chem. Res. Toxicol.* **2018**, 31, 350.）

例7-11：Since the doses of 1-MIM-OH varied, the data had to be normalized for a meaningful comparison. 1-MIM-GL administered in plant matrix formed 9 and 15 times more adducts in Hb and SA, respectively, than when it was tested as a purified compound. （*Arch. Toxicol.* **2019**, 93, 1515.）

例7-12：We have developed a strategy to generate cell-laden GelMA constructs with tunable and favorable microenvironments for various cell types by coaxial extrusion bioprinting of GelMA/alginate core/sheath microfibers, where the alginate sheath serves as a template to support and confine the GelMA hydrogel in the core to allow for subsequent UV crosslinking. （*Biofabrication* **2018**, 10, 024102.）

7.1.2　讨论部分的扩展

一旦开始讨论部分的撰写，就可很自然过渡到讨论的主体部分。此时应重点围绕研究结果中最能体现创新性或重要性的内容，从多个角度进行分析，解释数据背后蕴藏的规律或机制。撰写时务必反复锤炼，有理、有据、有条理地开展讨论，撰写质量与作者本人在此领域的知识储备水平、分析解决问题的能力密切相关。

撰写此部分时需要注意以下几点：

① 将研究结果与已有文献进行比较，清楚说明本研究与它们有何不同，对于不符合文献或者预期的结果应有合理的解释。

② 可以对之前结果做出新的解释，从而推动相关领域的进步。

③ 从实验设计、原理、分析方法、文献等多个角度，深入阐述研究结果，提出研究发现。

④ 推论要适度、科学并符合逻辑，避免提出研究数据支持不足的观点或结论。

⑤ 在探讨研究发现的重要性时，应实事求是，避免过度夸大。

⑥ 谨慎使用"For the first time"等类似的优先权声明，确保文献调研全面完整。

例7-13：Li et al. reported that the affinity of *N,N*-diethyl-type compounds for the H$^+$/OC antiporter is lower than that of *N,N*-dimethyl-type compounds due to steric hindrance. The present <u>study also showed that</u> uptake of amine A having the *N,N*-diethyl moiety was slower than that of diphenhydramine (Supplemental Fig. 2). （*J. Pharm. Sci.* **2021**, 110, 397.）

例7-14：<u>However</u>, 1 mmol/L TEA showed little inhibitory effect on the pregabalin uptake (Table Ⅲ). This result <u>is consistent with a previous report</u> that uptake of gabapentin, the substrate of both LAT1 andOCTN1, in hCMEC/D3 cells was hardly affected by any OCTN inhibitors, such as verapamil, amantadine, and corticosterone[10]. （*Pharm. Res.* **2018**, 35, 246.）

例7-15：<u>Interestingly</u>, the transporters involved in DON uptake differ in different cell types (Figs 3e and 4b), <u>possibly due to</u> the different expression levels of transporters in different tissues. OATPs are mainly expressed in intestinal cells and hepatocytes, whereas OCTs and OATs are mainly expressed in hepatocytes and kidney cells[33]. The differences in expression among the uptake transporters <u>may explain the differences</u> in the absorption, distribution and excretion of DON in different tissues. The over-expression of some potential transporters should be useful to identify which subtypes of these transporters are critical for DON uptake in future studies. （*Sci. Rep.* **2017**, 7, 5889.）

例7-16：The increased quantity of microvilli observed by us at the luminal side of ECs (Fig. 1B) also provides information about the vascular passage of fluid. This characteristic <u>has been reported by others</u> to be present in cerebral edemas of different origin, including ischemia and hypertension (Makarov et al., 2015; Lossinsky et al., 1995; Dietrich et al., 1984). （*Toxicology* **2018**, 408, 31.）

例7-17：Thirteen genes were completely absent from all the cells. Of these, BSEP, OATP-C and OATP 8 are known to be liver specific (Dean et al., 2001, Kim, 2003, Strautnieks et al., 1998), whereas OATP-F is predominantly expressed in brain and testes (Pizzagalli et al., 2002). OAT1 and 3 are kidney specific (Anzai et al., 2006). CAT3 is mainly expressed in thymus and other peripheral tissues (Vekony et al., 2001). Interestingly, PAT1, a proton-coupled amino acid transporter <u>which has been reported to be</u> expressed in Caco-2 cells (Chen et al., 2003) was not expressed in any of the cells in this study. （*Eur. J. Pharm. Sci.* **2008**, 35, 383.）

例7-18：<u>Despite multiple publications demonstrating</u> differences in immune response between men and women,[28–32] we did not find a sex-based difference in our study. <u>This may be due to</u> a smaller cohort size (*n*=98) than most of the prior studies. It may also reflect the fact that we are studying immune responses nearly 20 years after multiple doses of MMR vaccine, as waning immunity and/or repeated immunization may obscure any sex-based immune response differences. （*J. Thromb. Haemost.* **2020**, 18, 2613.）

7.1.3　讨论研究的局限性

任何科学研究都是在一定时间内完成的阶段性成果，受到科技发展、技术瓶颈、仪器条件等多重因素的限制，研究本身或多或少存在一定的局限性。讨论部分应告知读者此研究的局限性或不足之处，如有任何失败或矛盾的数据也应该提及，从而帮助读者正确地理解研究发现，也可能对他们自身的研究有所帮助。因此，讨论研究的局限性非常重要。

（1）解释自身工作的不足

在讨论自身工作不足时，可以说明研究的问题、当前知识理论、所用技术手段或者研究模型有何缺陷或瓶颈，也可以说明研究推论有何不足。

常用句型有：

It should be noted/mentioned that the present study is limited…

We concentrated/focused on only…

We have to point out that we do not…

Some limitations of this study are…

…is a limitation/ a serious drawback of this study.

…is not suitable for…

Our results are lack of…

The results do not imply…

Unfortunately/Regrettably,…

Although/However,….

解释自身工作不足的撰写范文如下。

例7-19：It should be mentioned that <u>our study is limited by</u> the fact that we used only one type of hepatic cells, the HepaRG cell lines, for the construction of 3DP-HOs, to demonstrate our proof of concept. （*Gut* **2021**, 70, 567.）

例7-20：In this study, putative N2-IS-dG was detected in traces, besides other till then unknown safrole-derived DNA adducts, <u>which were not analyzed in the present method</u> and may indicate again the low sensitivity compared to the NPL assay. （*Food Chem. Toxicol.* **2019**, 129, 424.）

例7-21：<u>However</u>, the use of immortalized cell lines <u>is a limitation</u> for hepatic study. Since primary human hepatocytes are difficult to seek and culture, alterative cell lines are still needed. （*Small* **2020**, 16, e1905505.）

例7-22：On one hand, this may due to the environmental or endogenous exposure of aldehydes. On the other hand, because individuals have different abilities to detoxify aldehydes and repair aldehyde-DNA adducts, the sample size ($n=32$) <u>may be too limited to</u> determining the potential differences between groups. （*J. Chromatogr. B Analyt. Technol. Biomed. Life Sci.* **2017**, 1060, 451.）

例7-23：Moreover, spheroid, organoid and engineered kidney cultures are not exposed to fluid shear stress, <u>unlike</u> the physiological renal lumen. These issues make spheroid and micro engineered cultures <u>not suitable for</u> high-throughput screening of drug-induced toxicity. （*Eur. J. Pharmacol.* **2016**, 790, 46.）

例7-24：Such 2D models have the advantage to be relatively simple and low in cost and form the basis of our current knowledge in cellular mechanisms. <u>However,</u> 2D cell cultures do not reproduce the *in vivo* microenvironment of the, which likely contributes to the functionally differentiated state of cells. (*Eur. J. Pharmacol.* **2016**, 790, 46.)

（2）说明研究局限性或负面数据可能产生的后果

说明研究局限性或负面数据可能产生的后果部分的撰写范文如下。

例7-25：Since we did not further investigate the absolute configuration of the found DNA adducts, we <u>could not clarify</u> if all four possible stereoisomers were formed (and these co-eluted), or if one enantiomeric pair (of one diastereomer), or a single adduct was formed. （*Food Chem. Toxicol.* **2018**, 116, 138.）

例7-26：<u>Another limitation</u> of the HepG2 cell line is that various nuclear receptors are expressed at a considerably lower level in these cells (Tolosa et al. 2016). Thus, compounds like phenobarbital, which acts via activation of CAR and PXR receptors, might not exhibit the complete toxicological feature compared to the in vivo situation. （*Arch. Toxicol.* **2018**, 92, 893.）

例7-27：Although amines E and G, which contain a morpholine ring, did not show temperature-dependence or trans-stimulation, the uptake of amine E was competitively inhibited by pyrilamine, and the K_i value was similar to the K_m value of pyrilamine uptake by hCMEC/D3 cells (19 mmol/L), as was also the case for amine D (Fig. 4). These results suggest the involvement of a pyrilamine-sensitive H^+/OC antiporter in uptake of amines E and G as well, though <u>it is not clear</u> whether the molecular species is the same as that involved in uptake of the other amines. Further studies are needed to clarify the reason for the difference. (*J. Pharm. Sci.* **110**, 397.)

例7-28：<u>Another limitation of the study is</u> the time frame studied. Our investigation was limited by the existing biospecimens and available participants and therefore focused on a narrow window of time 7 and 17 years after vaccination. It is possible that a fair amount of waning had already occurred before we recruited subjects, and the extremely low cellular immune responses that we detected (especially to mumps) support this hypothesis. (*J. Thromb. Haemost.* **2020**, 18, 2613.)

例7-29：As 3D cell culture techniques are increasingly asserted to improve cell culture translational relevance for toxicity screening, <u>few studies actually</u> compare critical phenotypic functional aspects of these models. <u>Lack of</u> phenotypic fidelity has been asserted to be <u>an important limitation</u> to the accuracy and predictability of *in vitro* cell-based toxicity assays. (*Pflugers. Arch.* **2018**, 470, 1311.)

（3）参考其他文献的类似问题

若参考其他文献的类似问题，该部分撰写范文如下。

例7-30：We demonstrated here that the anti-Xa activities measured using different reagents in the plasma from patients on UFH could vary up to 41%. <u>A similar pattern of results was already obtained</u> in plasmas spiked with UFH, even though differences were less significant than in patients' plasmas, probably because of limited commutability in materials as shown in samples used for quality control purposes in the case of aPTT for UFH monitoring.[38] Moreover, these <u>results were confirmed by</u> data obtained in the 2017 ECAT EQAP exercises. (*J. Thromb. Haemost.* **2020**, 18, 2613.)

例7-31：<u>A similar discrepancy was reported</u> in another study in South East Asia. In a study of 653 Vietnamese men and women, the prevalence of osteoporosis was 29% in women and 10% in men, with the local reference values. However, the prevalence was much higher −44% in women and 30% in men, when using the DXA-provided reference values[15]. (*BMC Musculoskelet. Disord.* **2020**, 21, 633.)

（4）写作技巧

在讨论研究局限性或者负面数据时，应采用诚实、明确的态度，同时也需要注意写作技巧，避免夸大研究不足，从而导致审稿人或者读者质疑甚至不认可研究发现。此外，指出研究不足之后，最好再次强调研究发现的正确性、重要性以及可能采取的补救措施，为别人或者自己的下一步研究打下伏笔。撰写时，可以尝试更加积极的表述方式。譬如，将下文中的例 7-32 换一种表达方式后，例 7-33 看起来就要积极许多。

例 7-32：The limitation of the present study is that the two animal experiments were not performed simultaneously. This will affect our results in terms of…

例 7-33：Although the two animal experiments were not conducted simultaneously, this will only affect our results in terms of …

例 7-33 通过以下方法减少了例 7-32 表述中的消极影响：

① "limitation" 不宜多次使用，以免读者不认同研究发现。如果必须多次提到，可以尝试使用 shortfall、shortcoming、pitfall、drawback、disadvantage 等同义词，减少可能产生的负面感受。

② 使用 "although" 和 "only" 等副词来修饰所说内容。"although" 告诉读者将有一些消极的言语，但是积极的话会随后出现。"only" 暗示影响有限，从而降低不足的严重程度。

③ 将两个句子合并为一个句子，减少读者思考消极内容的时间。

有助于减少消极程度的常用句型举例如下：

Although it is too early to draw statistically significant conclusions, …

Although at this time these answers cannot be given, …

However, more definite conclusions will be possible when…

Nevertheless, our study confirms that…

Despite this, the present study provides support for…

In any case, these results indicate that…

7.1.4 讨论部分的结束

可以按照下述方式结束讨论部分。

① 研究发现能否延伸到其他领域？如果可以，说明如何推广并提供必要的依据。

② 提出完善实验假说以及模型、设备等技术手段的方法。

③ 说明并解释是否忽略某些特定情况。

④ 承认因技术手段等方面的不足而导致目前无法提供的推论。

⑤ 重申选择论文主题的原因，使读者相信研究发现的正确性和重要性。

结束讨论部分的撰写范例如下。

例 7-34：Our untargeted wide-SIM/MS^2 scanning method in conjunction with targeted-MS^n are powerful approaches to screen for DNA adducts and <u>will be further employed to</u> advance our understanding of hazardous agents that form DNA adducts in the bladder and contribute to bladder carcinogenesis. （*Chem. Res. Toxicol.* **2018**, 31, 1382.）

例 7-35：This study also <u>provides a basis for</u> the integrated monitoring and assessing of exposure to toxins and could be used to investigate an individual's response to exposure to complex mixtures. （*Talanta* **2021**, 222, 121500.）

例 7-36：Moreover, a dietary questionnaire was not available, and thus, exposures to HAAs through the diet are uncertain. The measurements of urinary AA and HAA biomarkers, or possibly hair biomarkers for HAAs <u>would provide a better assessment of</u> meat consumption. （*Chem. Res. Toxicol.* **2018**, 31, 1382.）

例 7-37：<u>In summary</u>, we demonstrated a sensitive and reliable UPLC-MS/MS method to quantify dA-AAI adduct in DNA from human renal cell systems and tissue samples. We showed that RPTEC/TERT1 cells represented an appropriate model to investigate mechanism(s) underlying AAI-mediated DNA adduct formation in humans. In contrast, HEK293 may serve as excellent negative control to elucidate specific steps in metabolism of AAI in renal cells. （*Toxicology* **2019**, 420, 29.）

例 7-38：<u>Indeed</u>, the enhanced antitumour effect was confirmed by histological analysis, <u>revealing</u> an increased apoptosis and decreased proliferation in tumour xenografts treated with PPNP + FUS (Figure 7). Thus, our study <u>provides a new strategy to</u> efficiently and locally deliver drugs into the brain to treat glioma through combining FUS with PS-80-modification of nanoparticles. （*J. Cell. Mol. Med.* **2018**, 22, 4171.）

例 7-39：The current study did not address the mechanisms by which P-gp, MRP2, or CYP3A4 expression and/or activity are dysregulated in the intestine of pH rats. The pregnane X Receptor (PXR)-Retinoid X Receptor alpha stimulates

CYP3A4 transcription through the activation of the CYP3A4 promoter. P-gp is also regulated by nuclear receptors such as PXR[62], ERK-FOXO 3a, while MRP2 is regulated by protein kinase C, radixin, nuclear factor kB, human cAMP response element-binding protein, and the CAATT box enhancer binding protein. Further studies are planned to investigate the molecular mechanism underlying the alteration in drug efflux transporters and detoxifying enzymes associated with pH. （*BMC Gastroenterol.* **2021**, 21, 2.）

例7-40：A further area which merits exploration is the quantitative relationship between metabolite changes in this *in vitro* setting and results observed in animal studies. Is there a possibility to distinguish between true adverse effects and adaptive changes at the level of metabolites? Can quantitative differences in the sensitivity of humans and rats (as the most commonly used animal model) also be seen when comparing rat and human cells when applying metabolomics to liver cells of both species? Although at this time these answers cannot be given, they become testable with the technology presented in this paper. （*Arch. Toxicol.* **2018**, 92, 893.）

7.1.5 讨论部分的写作质量评估

当完成讨论部分的写作时，可以围绕"如何进行研究"以及"如何分析研究发现"，参考下列清单进行核对，以评估论文部分的写作质量。

① 是否对本文重要发现及其重要性进行了客观的陈述和解释？

② 是否对实验结果进行了科学合理的解释，而不是实验结果的简单复述？

③ 文中所有推论是否都有数据和图表的支持？

④ 实验结果有无其他可能的解释？

⑤ 是否有效区分了事实与推测？

⑥ 有无隐藏任何不利或者不符合预期的实验数据或意外结果？

⑦ 是否对负面数据或与文献报道矛盾之处做出了合理的解释？

⑧ 有无对实验数据进行过度解读，从而得出不可信的结论？

⑨ 是否明确说明实验结果与假说之间的关系（支持或拒绝）？是否产生了新的理论或假说？

⑩ 讨论撰写是否简明扼要、切中主题？

⑪ 在文献引用、数据选取等方面，能否确保研究没有明显的偏见？

⑫ 是否根据前言内容讨论了研究发现？

⑬ 是否将本研究与已有文献相结合，以解释新发现或新结果，并比较两者之间的优劣？

⑭ 对文献的批判是合理并有建设性的吗？

⑮ 是否说明了研究局限性，并提供了合理的解释？

7.1.6 讨论部分的写作范例

下文以 2021 年发表的一篇题为 "Investigating PEGDA and GelMA Microgel Models for Sustained 3D Heterotypic Dermal Papilla and Keratinocyte Co-Cultures" 的论文（*Int. J. Mol. Sci.* **2021**, 22, 2143.）为例，展示讨论的构架与写法。

①In this paper, we demonstrated two possible combinations of culturing epithelial (i.e., HaCaT keratinocytes) and dermal cells (i.e., DP) in PEGDA and GelMA microwells. For PEGDA microwells, it was observed that both cell types exhibited relatively low attachment to the gel surfaces, resulting in the initial aggregation of DP cells followed by the HaCaT keratinocytes to yield a core-shell configuration. On the contrary, it was observed that DP cells were adherent towards GelMA surfaces, hence forming a layer on the walls and the base of the microwells 24 h post-seeding. ［第一段开头简要介绍研究发现：HaCaT 角质形成细胞及真皮毛乳头细胞（DP）可在 PEGDA 微孔中可形成核壳结构的球样体。相反，DP 细胞黏附在 GelMA 表面。］②A similar configuration was attempted by Pan et al., whereby the mesenchymal cells [i.e., human dermal fibroblasts (HDF)] were compartmentalized within the PEGDA hydrogel scaffold while the epithelial cells (i.e., HaCaT) were seeded into the microwells made from HDF-encapsulated PEGDA hydrogels[13]. However, the difference between these two models lies in the availability of the mesenchymal component to interact with the HaCaT keratinocytes. The mesenchymal component in Pan's model (i.e., HDF) would have been more restricted as cells were encapsulated within the gel as compared to our current model where the mesenchymal component (i.e., DP cells) was directly coating the base and the walls of the GelMA microwells, due to its adhesive nature towards the surfaces. （将本研究所用细胞培养模型与已经发表的文献进行了比较，讨论了所用模型之间的区别。）③When cultured over prolonged duration (i.e., up to 10 days), we observed that the sizes of the heterotypic spheroids within PEGDA microwells were reduced drastically, while the sizes of the aggregates within GelMA microwells remained relatively constant. （随后描述研究中发现的现象：当培养时间长达 10 天时，PEGDA 微孔内异型球体的大小急剧减小， 而 GelMA 微孔内聚集体大小保持相对恒定。下一段将对此展开讨论。）

① We hypothesized that the reduction in the sizes of the co-cultures within PEGDA microwells was mainly attributed to the exfoliation of HaCaT keratinocytes, owning to their overall poor intercellular adhesion, as reported in previous literature [15,16]. （根据现有文献，提出对此现象的假说：PEGDA 微孔内共培养物尺寸的减少主要归因于 HaCaT 角质形成细胞的脱落。） ②Therefore, we decided to investigate the behavior of HaCaT keratinocyte inside both PEGDA and GelMA microwells. （解释研究思路。） ③As expected（果不其然，用此短语告诉读者下面的实验结果符合实验假说）, the HaCaT aggregates reduced in size as the HaCaT keratinocytes exfoliated and left the microwells after 10 days of culture within the PEGDA microwells. Little changes were observed inside the GelMA microwells containing only HaCaT keratinocytes. We hypothesized that the HaCaT keratinocytes remained within the microwells, due to better attachment. …

……（分段详述研究发现及其意义。）

For future studies, immunofluorescence can be used to explore the influence of more morphogens, including Wnt10A, Wnt10B, and Shh on *in vitro* models for hair follicular engineering. In addition, the concentrations of PEGDA and GelMA in the hydrogels can be varied to study their potential effects on DP-HaCaT interactions. （最后一段对将来工作进行展望。）

7.2 结论的写作

结论（Conclusions）是作者对实验假设支持与否、研究结果、重要发现以及可能的推广应用所做出的总结性陈述，一般在论文主体内容的最后一段，作为讨论或整篇文章的结尾。一些期刊中，讨论中的最后一段作为结论。然而，更多的期刊明确要求有单独的结论部分。《南村辍耕录》中所述，"作乐府亦有法，曰凤头、猪肚、豹尾六字是也"。一篇好的论文，应有点明中心、提升高度、注入灵魂的"豹尾"。作为论文的收尾部分，结论是概括要点和突出价值的最后机会，很有可能是审稿人或读者用来判定这篇文章的最后依据。因此，结论必须清晰明了，能够突出论文的精华，并通过建议、影响和潜在应用等叙述增加论文的价值，从而给人留下良好印象。

需要留意的是，结论不是对文章的简单总结，不要从摘要（Abstraction）、前言（Introduction）和讨论（Discussion）中重复完全相同的内容。在写作中应做到结论鲜明，直截了当，主题升华，突出论文之立意，拔高文章之主题。一般而言，药学论文的结论部分为一至两段，包含以下一项或多项内容。

① 简要回顾研究中最重要的发现，指出这些发现如何推动相关领域的发展，以及能否推广到其他领域。

例7-41：This study <u>provides the basis for future method development</u> to study multiple alkylation DNA adducts, and approaches for genotoxic impurities risk and cancer risk evaluations. （*J. Pharm. Biomed. Anal.* **2019**, 166, 387.）

例7-42：These results confirm that the investigated turkey and chicken *in vivo* models can be used interchangeably and are <u>valuable alternatives to</u> animal models as a tool for genotoxicity assessment, e.g. for regulatory purposes. （*Food Chem. Toxicol.* **2019,** 129, 424.）

例7-43：<u>To our knowledge, our study is the first report to</u> identify a DNA adduct of a cooked mutagen in human prostate by a specific LC-MS measurement. A significant percentage of prostate cancer patients harbor dG-C8-PhIP. （*Anal. Chem.* **2016**, 88, 12508.）

例7-44：Compared to other MALDI MS platforms (e.g., MALDI Orbitrap MS), the developed method allows for mass measurements of polysaccharides at a higher resolving power in a larger *m/z*-range. We envision broader applicability of this analytical approach with applications ranging from the biopharma (e.g., analysis of glycoconjugate vaccines and heparins) to the food industry (e.g., analysis of pectin). （*Anal. Chem.* **2021**, 93, 4666.）

例 7-45：The experimental results <u>provided a basis for</u> the determination of Aconitum alkaloids, <u>paving way for</u> the clinical application of Aconitum and its extracts. （*ACS Pharmacol. Transl. Sci.* **2020**, 4, 118.）

例 7-46：<u>Notably</u>, this approach could potentially be adapted to detect any analyte as long as antibody directed against it is available. Thus, <u>we anticipate that</u> the technology will be particularly useful for the detection of other clinically relevant molecules as a versatile tool. (*Talanta* **2021**, 224, 121921.)

例 7-47：<u>All the above results indicated that</u> the novel material would be a promising adsorbent, and the proposed method <u>has good potential on</u> the trace contaminant analysis in aqueous samples. (*Talanta* **2021**, 225, 121846.)

例 7-48：<u>In future studies</u>, the DNA trapping method described for measuring reactive metabolites from a PAH can be adapted for other chemicals, as well as in screening for genotoxic metabolites as part of a procedure for risk assessment of environmental contaminants. (J. Chromatogr. B Analyt. *Technol. Biomed. Life Sci.* **2020**, 1152, 122276.)

② 结合研究的局限性，给出进一步完善研究的建议。

例 7-49：<u>Due to</u> the weak sampling level, these findings <u>must be confirmed on</u> a larger cohort. It will be important to consolidate the use of these profiles of exocyclic DNA adducts as specific biomarkers of systemic exposure to aldehydes present in various environments. （*Toxicol. Lett.* **2020**, 331, 57.）

例 7-50：The formaldehyde detection scheme designed in this paper <u>has the characteristics of</u> low cost, portability, rapid detection, high selectivity and sensitivity. This method can only detect one sample at a time in the process of implementation, thus, <u>it will be improved towards</u> the high-through put multi-objective application mode in the subsequent study. <u>In future, the method will be promising for</u> the rapid quantitative detection of trace formaldehyde in various other substances. （*Food Chem.* **2021**, 340, 127930.）

例 7-51：Considering that the matrices of aquatic products generally suffer from the interference of gentamicin, <u>future works should</u> collect water and sediment samples from an aquiculture area to determine the effect of gentamicin on environment. <u>Furthermore</u>, the occurrence of artificial addition must be determined based on the concentration of gentamicin both in aquatic product and its survival environment to ensure food safety. （*J. Chromatogr. B Analyt. Technol. Biomed. Life Sci.* **2018**, 1093, 167.）

例7-52：<u>Currently, this method is limited by</u> the spot size of the robotic spotter to a spatial resolution of approximately 250 μm. Robotic spotters having reduced droplet sizes and improved deposition accuracies will <u>provide better resolution for</u> future imaging experiments. Different tissues must also be explored in which there are multiple microenvironments (kidneys, brains, etc.) within a single tissue that may cause differential extraction and/or ionization of the analytes of interest. （*Anal. Chem.* **2016**, 88, 2392.）

例7-53：This study did not <u>investigate the mechanism behind</u> the effects of anticoagulant type on plasma lipids though several potential explanations have been proposed. <u>Further studies should be directed toward</u> understanding the mechanism behind the differential anticoagulant effects, temperature effects, and storage effects on plasma lipids and metabolites. （*Biomolecules* **2019**, 9, 200.）

例7-54：Current knowledge of drug-host interactions in PM-DILI <u>is still limited</u>. More valuable biomarkers need to be discovered and validated for accurate PM-DILI diagnosis and prediction. （*Acta Pharmacol. Sin.* **2021**, 42, 27.）

③ 研究者的下一步研究计划。

例7-55：The method was successfully applied to a murine pharmacokinetic study that provided previously unavailable data into the role of CYP3A-mediated metabolism as a pathway of vincristine elimination. Our ongoing studies will <u>employ the method to gain mechanistic insights into</u> the role of vincristine metabolism in drug-drug interactions and to identify additional sources of inter-individual pharmacokinetic variability associated with vincristine-induced peripheral neuropathy. （*J. Chromatogr. B.* **2021**, 1168, 122591.）

例7-56：This study could support that the pharmacological and medicinal properties of Ephedra alata may not linked to one or a few of its constituents, but sometimes to the interaction of plant molecules. <u>Further research is in progress in our laboratory to</u> explore the effect of ME on antitumor activity of cisplatin. （*Environ. Sci. Pollut Res. Int.* **2020**, 27, 12792.）

例7-57：<u>In the future, we will further</u> incorporate *in vitro* mechanistic data that influence hepatotoxicity, such as metabolizing enzymes, liver transporters, and various pathway profiles, to improve risk assessment for hepatotoxicity. （*Mol. Pharm.* **2019**, 16, 393.）

例7-58：<u>Further studies are necessary to </u>determine whether commonly used cationic drugs or herbs containing cationic components may cause transporter-medicated drug-drug interactions in clinical practice.（*J. Ethnopharmacol.* **2020**, 252, 112581.）

例7-59：Our observations can be used to develop strategies for minimising acylation and for investigating the biological properties of leuprorelin-loaded PLGA formulations. <u>We are also working on</u> stability of leuprorelin microspheres following incubation under *in vitro* and *in vivo* conditions, which will be the subject of a next publication. （*Int. J. Pharm.* **2019**, 560, 273.）

7.2.1 结论与摘要的区别

不可避免地，结论和摘要之间会有一些重叠的内容，都会指出研究的主要内容并点明重要发现。但结论区别于摘要，因为此部分是针对那些对本研究有兴趣并掌握了相关专业知识的读者，通过阅读论文的前面部分，对文中的关键概念也有了深入了解。从写作角度考虑，结论与摘要、引言相比，更为简短精悍，在内容上需要注意以下几点：

① 对背景知识不再赘述；
② 对研究中的发现进行重点说明；
③ 简述讨论部分尚未涉及的局限性；
④ 简述潜在应用价值或后续研究。

下面以一篇题为"Formic Acid of ppm Enhances LC-MS/MS Detection of UV Irradiation-Induced DNA Dimeric Photoproducts"的论文（*Anal. Chem.* **2020**, 92, 1197.）为例，比较摘要与结论的区别。

摘要：① Cyclobutane pyrimidine dimers (CPDs) and pyrimidine (6-4) pyrimidone photoproducts (6-4PPs) are genotoxic DNA lesions and mainly generated on thymine-thymine (T-T) dinucleotides upon UV irradiation.

Regarding the sensitivity, specificity, and accuracy of analytical methods, it is of first choice to develop a reliable assay for simultaneous detection of these DNA lesions using liquid chromatography-tandem mass spectrometry (LC-MS/MS). （简要介绍课题背景和研究意义。）②However, the dilemma is the low detection sensitivity of the phosphate-containing dimeric photoproducts even using most favorable negative-ion mode for LC-MS/MS analysis. （指出当前存在的问题。）③Unexpectedly, we observed that the detection sensitivity of T-T CPD and 6-4PP could be significantly improved using formic acid/acetic acid (~ppm) as an additive of the mobile phase for reversed-phase LC-MS/MS analysis. This is the first demonstration of the enhancement of LC-MS/MS signals by formic acid/acetic acid in negative-ion mode. Of note, these acidic agents are often used for positive-ion mode in LC-MS assays. Benefited from the developed method, we could quantify both T-T CPD and 6-4PP in mouse embryonic stem cells upon UVC irradiation at low dosage. （介绍作者采用的方法以及重要发现。）④ This sensitive method is applicable to the screening and identification of genes involved in formation, signaling, and repair of UV lesion. （表明该研究的应用价值。）。

结论：① This work demonstrated that the LC-MS detection of CPD and 6-4PP dinucleoside monophosphates could be greatly enhanced by formic acid of ppm as an additive. （没有背景介绍，首句就总结论文的主要内容和重要发现。） ② By the application of the developed method, CPD and 6-4PP were sensitively detected and accurately quantified in mES cells upon UVC irradiation at low dosage. （高度凝练研究发现的具体应用。） ③ It is expected that the presented approach should be extended for LC-MS/MS detection of other UV-induced dimeric photoproducts or DNA lesions containing a monophosphate moiety. （扩展本研究的应用领域。）

7.2.2　结论的写作质量评估

当完成结论部分的写作时，可参考以下要点评估该部分的写作质量。

① 时态与语法是否正确？一般过去时用于描述所做研究、重申研究结果、解释本次研究发现，一般现在时则用于解释客观事实、比较研究结

果以及概括研究发现。

　　② 结论是否是前文的简单重复？结论与摘要、引言和讨论的最后一段有无足够的区分度？

　　③ 结论的长度是否合适（通常不超过 1 至 2 段）？

　　④ 关于实验方法或者过程，是否最多只给一句解释（一般不需要在结论中说明）？

　　⑤ 结论是否做到了论断鲜明、表述简单明了？

　　⑥ 结论是否有实验数据的充分支持？科学性是否无误？

　　⑦ 结论是否有亮点且有重要意义？

　　⑧ 结论所提出建议是否合理？可能的应用是否可行？

　　⑨ 是否介绍了研究的潜在价值及影响？

课后练习与讨论

1. 讨论部分的撰写过程中应该注意哪些事项？
2. 根据范例，尝试将讨论的写作技巧运用到自己的论文写作中。
3. 如何确保讨论部分的写作质量？
4. 结论部分在写作中应该包含哪些内容？
5. 结论与摘要之间的区别有哪些，为什么会有这些区别？
6. 结论部分的写作中会用到哪些时态？并分析几篇文献中关于结论部分的写作技巧。

第 8 章　•○

实验方法与补充材料

8.1　实验方法的写作

8.1.1　实验方法的写作要求和技巧

　　实验方法（Experimental Methods）是指描述实验过程中所使用的试剂、耗材、仪器、实验动物和研究人群等，以及用其进行研究的方法。实验方法这个部分通常有几种不同的表述方式，包括 Methods、Methods and Materials、Experimental Section、Method Description 等。在某种程度上，实验方法的写作要足够详细，让他人很容易按照所提供的材料和方法进行实验，并且能够达到较好的重现性。在药学专业论文中，该部分的首段通常会包括：①实验所用材料从何处获得，或者采用什么方式获得；②材料的质量和纯度通过何种方式鉴定评估；③概括说明论文中的一些基本方法；④特殊实验的实验场地和基本规则等。以下列文献（*Nature* **2010**，468，1067.）的 METHODS SUMMARY 为例。

METHODS SUMMARY

　　The inhibitor JQ1 was synthesized in both racemic and enantiomerically pure format using the synthetic route outlined in scheme 1 and scheme 2 (Supplementary Methods) and its structure was fully characterized. Human bromodomains were expressed in bacteria as His-tagged proteins and were purified by nickelaffinity and gel-filtration chromatography. Protein integrity was assessed by SDS-PAGE and electro-spray mass spectrometry on an Agilent 1100 Series LC/MSD TOF. All crystallizations were carried out at 4℃ using the sitting-drop vapour-diffusion method. X-ray diffraction data were collected at the Swiss Light source beamline X10SA, or using a Rigaku FR-E generator. Structures were determined by molecular replacement. Isothermal titration calorimetry experiments were performed at 15℃ on a VP-ITC titration microcalorimeter (MicroCal). Thermal melting experiments were carried out on an Mx3005p RT-PCR machine (Stratagene) using SYPRO Orange as a fluorescence probe. Dose-ranging small-molecule studies of proliferation were performed in white, 384-well plates (Corning) in DMEM media containing 10% FBS. Compounds were delivered with a JANUS pin-transfer robot and proliferation measurements weremade onanEnvisionmultilabel platereader (PerkinElmer). Murine xenografts were established by injecting NMC cells in 30% Matrigel (BD Biosciences) into the flank of 6-week-old female NCr nude mice (Charles River Laboratories). Tumour measurements were assessed by caliper measurements, and volume was calculated using the formula Vol50.53L3W2. All mice were humanely killed, and tumours were fixed in 10% formalin for histopathological examination. Quantitative immunohistochemistry was performed using the Aperio Digital Pathology Environment (Aperio Technologies) at the DF/HCC Core Laboratory at the Brigham and Women's Hospital.

　　实验方法的写作相对来说是比较简单的，也经常是论文手稿中最先完成的部分。为了更好地完成该部分的写作，一个关键技能是要写得非常清晰，注意语句间的逻辑关系，确保一个句子不超过两个步骤或实验操作，使读者很容易跟随文中的描述。另一个关键的技巧是确保描述的完整性，不能因为步骤的缺失导致读者出现理解偏差或实验重复失败；同时，也可通过引用已知文献中的相同或类似方法，使该部分保持尽可能的简洁。下面这个例子（*J. Med. Chem.* **2014**, 57, 8249.）就很好地体现了完整性和简洁性的完美统一，并且描述也足够清晰。

Cellular Assays. Cellular phosphorylation and proliferation assays were performed as reported previously by ourselves.[6]

***In Vivo* Antitumor Efficacy Studies.** All *in vivo* efficacy studies were performed as reported previously by ourselves.[6]

Rat *in Vivo* Toxicology Studies. Studies were carried out in accordance with U.K. Home Office legislation (Animals [Scientific Procedures] Act 1986) and AstraZeneca's institutional policies. The animals used were 10-week-old male RccHan:WIST rats obtained from Harlan, U.K. Animals (n=3/compound) received a single oral dose of compound as a suspension in 0.5% *W/V* HPMC/0.1% *W/V* Tween in deionized water at a concentration of 20 mg/mL. Blood glucose levels were measured using an Accuchek Active meter (ACCU-CHEK Active; Roche, Basel, Switzerland). Serum insulin concentrations were determined using a commercial rat ELISA kit (Mercodia, Upsala, Sweden). Water and food were available ad libitum.

在实验方法部分的写作中，一般会遵循"基本、简洁、没有结论"的规则。药学专业论文中的实验方法通常包括以下一项或几项：

① 药物分子及中间体的详细合成方法和分离鉴定方法；

② 化合物的体外和体内生物活性测试方法；

③ 化合物的理化性质测试方法；

④ 化合物的药物代谢动力学测试方法；

⑤ 化合物的体外和体内的选择性、毒性测试方法；

⑥ 药物在不同研究体系中的分析测试方法；

⑦ 其他相关方法。

8.1.2　实验方法的写作范例

例8-1：药物分子合成路线的实验方法写作（*J. Med. Chem.* **2014**，57，2033.；已获授权许可，版权所有©2014，美国化学会）

药物分子 Ledipasvir（**39**）是经过多步反应获得，以从化合物 **39a** 合成化合物 **39b** 为例，文中所描述的实验方法包含以下内容：

① 产物的完整化学命名（文中编号）；

② 所用的材料和反应参数：反应试剂（用量）、溶剂（用量）、温度、时间等；

③ 反应操作的方法及注意事项；

④ 监控反应的方法；

⑤ 后处理及分离纯化的方法；

⑥ 实验结果：产量和收率、产物性状、产物结构表征。

化合物的结构表征时应注意以下几点：

① 每个化合物须有正确的化学命名；

② 每个化合物须有全文唯一的编号；

③ 固体化合物须有熔点信息，如为非全新结构，则必须给出参考文献；

④ 全新结构的目标产物，须同时给出核磁共振氢谱图（^{1}H NMR）和碳谱（^{13}C NMR）信息；

⑤ 目标产物须给出纯度信息；

(a) *N*-Fluorobenzenesulfonimide, KHMDS, THF; (b) *i*-PrMgCl, 2-chloro-*N*-methoxy-*N*-methylacetamide, THF; (c) **12** K₂CO₃, KI, acetone; (d) NH₄OAc, PhMe; (e) **38a**, Pd(OAc)₂, PPh₃, NaHCO₃, DME/H₂O; (f) HCl/dioxane/DCM; (g) **11**, HATU, *i*-Pr₂NEt, DMF.

⑥ 目标产物须给出质谱鉴定结果，注明分子离子峰。

其中的核磁共振谱图（NMR）解析和写作要点：

① 给出谱种、仪器分辨率、溶剂信息。例如：¹H NMR (300 MHz,

DMSO-d_6) δ 等。

② 化学位移由大到小，从低场到高场排列。

③ 氢谱信号的撰写格式：化学位移（峰型，偶合常数，积分数值，信号归属）。例如：3.64 (dd, $J = 6.0$ Hz, 2H, —CH$_2$NH—)。

④ 碳谱只需给出化学位移信息，无需对各组峰进行具体归属。

2-Bromo-9,9-difluoro-7-iodo-9*H*-fluorene (39b). 2-Bromo-7-iodo-9*H*-fluorene (39a, 705 mg, 1.90 mmol) and NFSI (1.80 g, 5.70 mmol) were dissolved in THF (9.5 mL) and cooled to −20℃. KHMDS (1.0 mol/L in THF, 5.7 mL, 5.7 mmol) was added dropwise over 9 min. On completion of the addition, the reaction mixture was warmed to 0℃. After an additional 80 min at 0℃, TLC indicated completion of the reaction, and excess base was quenched by addition of MeOH (30 drops) followed by hexane (20 mL). The suspension was filtered over Celite and concentrated. The resulting residue was dissolved in 20% DCM/hexane (20 mL) (some solid does not dissolve) and passed over a short silica plug. The plug was rinsed with hexane (～170 mL) until TLC indicated all desired product was eluted. The liquid was concentrated to provide 2-bromo-9,9-difluoro-7-iodo-9*H*-fluorene **39b** (626 mg, 81% yield) as a pale-yellow-orange solid. The material is essentially pure by NMR and LCMS. ^{1}H NMR (CDCl$_3$) δ 7.94 (1H, d, $J = 1.2$ Hz), 7.81 (1H, d, $J = 7.8$ Hz), 7.74 (1H, d, $J = 1.4$ Hz), 7.60 (1H, d, $J = 8.3$ Hz), 7.41 (1H, d, $J = 8.1$ Hz), 7.29 (1H, d, $J = 8.0$ Hz). ^{19}F NMR (CDCl$_3$) δ − 111.034 (2F, s).

在药物分子合成路线的写作中，还需注意以下几点：

① 每个非商业可得的化合物，其合成方法一般都必须写出，不能出现有化合物而无合成描述的情况。

② 在某些情况下，一些简单的已知化合物可以不必提供合成方法，但要其合成方法的参考文献。

③ 如果多个化合物的合成方法路线相同，可写一个通用的合成路线（general procedure A）并引用指明。

④ 其中涉及的一些专业术语的格式需要注意，如核磁结果中的化学位移 δ 需要斜体等。

例 8-2：体内药效学的实验方法写作（*J. Med. Chem.* **2017**，60，8369.；已获授权许可，版权所有©2017，美国化学会）

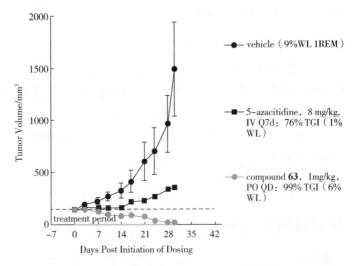

Figure 7. Kasumi-1 mouse xenograft study with compound **63**. Values represent mean±SE (*n*=8/group); WL=maximum mean weight loss; REM=removed from study due to morbidity.

The tumor xenograft study was conducted at CrownBio, Inc. (Beijing, China). Female NOD.SCID mice (HFK Bioscience Co., Ltd., Beijing, China) were *γ*-irradiated (200 rads) 24 hours before receiving a right flank subcutaneous inoculation of 10 million Kasumi-1 cells (ATCC) in 0.2 mL of 1∶1 PBS:matrigel (BD Biosciences, CA). Daily administration of compound or vehicle was initiated at the time of size match randomization (8 per group) when the mean tumor volume reached approximately 250 mm^3 and continued until study endpoint (mean tumor volume of controls reaches 1500 mm^3). The tumors were measured by a pair of calipers twice a week and tumor volumes were calculated according to the formula $V=L\times W^2/2$ (*V*: volume, mm^3; *L*: length, mm. *W*: width, mm). Tumor growth inhibition, TGI%=100−mean tumor volume of treatment group / mean tumor volume of control group×100.

与实验结果的写作不同，实验方法的描述尽量客观重现实验材料、操作和所用方法，对结果不做解释说明，同时必须清晰完整地描述以下几项内容：

① 实验是在哪开展的，用了哪些动物，每组包含多少只动物？动物实验是否符合伦理规范？

② 具体的给药方式和用药时间。

③ 肿瘤体积和肿瘤生长抑制率（TGI）的测定方法。

8.1.3　实验方法写作的时态语态

实验方法部分通常采用被动语态，用一般过去时进行写作。

① 被动语态在实验方法部分的写作中是一种既必要又恰当的方式，这是因为该部分的重点是要描述做了什么，而无需强调是谁做的。

② 用一般过去时也是显而易见的，这是因为实验方法中所描述的是过去发生的事情。此外，一般过去时也有助于将研究中所做的事情与他人所做的事情区分开来（用一般现在时）。

8.2　补充材料的写作

虽然不同期刊的篇幅不尽相同，但对正文的篇幅总是会做出限制。为了避免论文正文部分的篇幅过长，通常会将相关实验的支持性与辅助性数据、结果、方法等写入论文的补充材料中，也就是所谓的"Supporting Information（SI）"。补充材料单独排版，通常会将其链接提供在对应论文的网络页面或者论文的文末中，一般可免费下载。对很多期刊来说，补充材料并不是必需的，但一般建议提供，以增加研究数据和方法的可信度。

例8-3：通过论文的网络主页找到 Supporting Information

RETURN TO ISSUE　　〈 PREV　　**ARTICLE**　　NEXT 〉

Discovery and Biological Evaluation of a Novel Highly Potent Selective Butyrylcholinsterase Inhibitor

Qi Li, Shuaishuai Xing, Ying Chen, Qinghong Liao, Baichen Xiong, Siyu He, Weixuan Lu, Yang Liu, Hongyu Yang, Qihang Li, Feng Feng, Wenyuan Liu, Yao Chen*, and Haopeng Sun*

Cite this: *J. Med. Chem.* 2020, 63, 17, 10030–10044

Publication Date: July 28, 2020 ∨

https://doi.org/10.1021/acs.jmedchem.0c01129

Copyright © 2020 American Chemical Society

RIGHTS & PERMISSIONS　✔ Subscribed

Article Views　　　Altmetric　　　Citations

1097　　　　　　　7　　　　　　5

LEARN ABOUT THESE METRICS

Share　Add to　Export

PDF (5 MB)　　　SI Supporting Info (1) »　　　SUBJECTS: Rodent models, inhibitors, ∨

Journal of Medicinal Chemistry

■ ASSOCIATED CONTENT

⑤ Supporting Information

The Supporting Information is available free of charge at
https://pubs.acs.org/doi/10.1021/acs.jmedchem.0c01129.

Basic information and target inhibitory activities of the
13 hit compounds; binding mode with *h*BChE and
alignment of binding mode with donepezil in *h*AChE of
8012−9656; structural spectrum data of intermediates,
final compounds (**8012−9656**) and tacrine; molecular
formula strings of all compounds; everyday body weight
of mice in the acute toxicity assay; standard curve of the
mouse $A\beta_{1-42}$ ELISA kit (PDF)

不同杂志对补充材料的要求不同，有些杂志要求需要在正文最后写明补充材料中所包含的内容。

例8-4：通过论文的文末提供的超链接获取 Supporting Information

nature chemical biology

ARTICLE

PUBLISHED ONLINE: 10 JUNE 2015 | DOI: 10.1038/NCHEMBIO.1858

Catalytic *in vivo* protein knockdown by small-molecule PROTACs

Additional information

Supplementary information and chemical compound information is available in the
online version of the paper. Reprints and permissions information is available online at
http://www.nature.com/reprints/index.html. Correspondence and requests for materials
should be addressed to I.C. or C.M.C.

根据不同杂志的要求，实验方法的一部分或全部可以出现在正文中。一般而言，重要的实验方法写在正文中，次要的实验方法写在补充材料中。实验方法如果作为正文的一部分，一般以文本表述为主，格式较为规范。

补充材料的格式比较多样，包括 PDF 或 Word 文本、Excel 表格、图片、图形、音频、视频等。内容可以是中间体的合成方法、化合物的晶体结构数据、体内的药代动力学数据、各种谱图（^{1}H NMR、^{13}C NMR、LC、LC-MS）等。

例8-5：化合物的结构表征谱图（氢谱、碳谱、质谱和纯度信息）

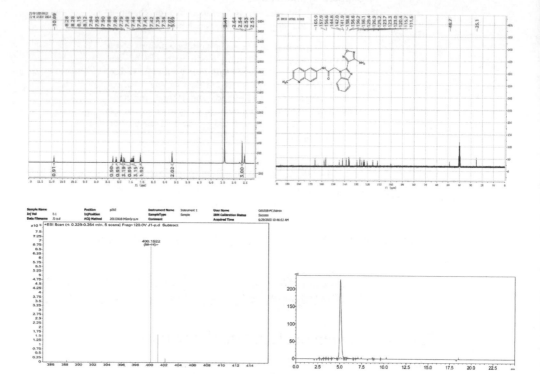

例8-6：Supporting information 中的表格

Table S1. Selectivity profile of I-BET151, iBET-BD1, iBET-BD2 and GSK620 determined by TR-FRET assay.

	FRET IC$_{50}$ (nmol/L) Mean±SEM (n)			
	I-BET151	iBET-BD1	iBET-BD2	GSK620
BRD2 BD1	7±31 (16)	75±4 (6).	10965 (1)[a]	25420±2591 (13)[d]
BRD3 BD1	37±13 (15)	41+5 (6)	36317±1182 (2)[b]	25802±6171 (6)[e]
BRD4 BD1	36±6 (16)	41±3 (16)	70558±51783 (3)[c]	17442± 1857 (14)
BRDT BD1	119±4 (16)	143±14 (6)	>50119 (8)	22634±2353 (9)[f]
BRD2 BD2	274±36 (16)	3950±290 (8)	264±53 (9)	285±20 (20)
BRD3 BD2	87±8 (16)	1210±65 (6)	98±6 (8)	72±4 (16)
BRD4 BD2	329±22 (16)	5843±304 (16)	49±4 (12)	81±9 (16)
BRDT BD2	1680±169 (16)	17451±1938 (6)	214±53 (8)	184 19 (18)

a. also tested>501 19 (n=10); b. also tested>50119 (n=6); c. also tested>50119 (n=8); d. also tested>50119 (n=8); e. also tested>501 19 (n=10); f. also tested>50119 (n=7) plus>16596 (n=2).

8.3　实验方法和补充材料的写作质量评估

当完成实验方法和补充材料的写作时，认真核对以下问题，以评估该部分的写作质量以及数据的准确无误。

① 是否查看过对应期刊中关于这部分的内容、格式规范、数字使用、图片要求等的指南？

② 所提供的实验方法是否准确可靠？是否已经涵盖了所有步骤？有没有遗漏或表述不清？

③ 是否以一种读者易于理解的方式描述了实验方法，使他们能够重复文中所述的工作？

④ 每个句子是否包含适当数量的可操作步骤？

⑤ 是否做到了尽可能的简洁？对于已知文献中相同或类似的实验方法，有没有通过引用相关文献避免不必要的重复描述？

⑥ 实验方法的描述是否正确地使用了时态和语态？

⑦ 谱图是否含有杂质峰？跟文献报道中的数据是否一致？

⑧ 图片是否足够清晰？

8.4　实验方法和补充材料部分的常见句型表达

实验方法和补充材料部分的常见句型有：

① Nuclear magnetic resonance (NMR) spectra were recorded on Bruker 400 MHz spectrometer.

② LC/MS was conducted on a Thermo Finnigan MSQ Std and a Dionex Summit HPLC System (model P680A HPG) equipped with a Gemini 5 μm C18 110A column (30 mm Å～4.60 mm), eluting with solvent A and solvent B.

③ Pharmacokinetic studies were performed in male Sprague-Dawley(SD) rats.

④ THP-1 cells (ATCC) were cultured in RPMI (1640＋10%) FBS and were grown at 37℃ with 5% CO_2.

⑤ The statistical significance of differences in protein fold change was calculated using a *z*-test with a robust estimation of the standard deviation and calculating the *P* values for all measurements.

⑥ Mice were sacrificed five hours after final dose.

⑦ All experiments were conducted under an approved protocol.

⑧ Cells were plated either in 96-well plates or 6-well plates 24 h before transfection with short interfering RNA (siRNA).

⑨ The Annexin Ⅴ-FITC Apoptosis Detection Kit Ⅰ (BD Biosciences) was used to detect apoptotic cells.

⑩ The reaction mixture was stirred at $-78\,^{\circ}\text{C}$ for 30 min and then warmed to room temperature.

⑪ Metabolic stability *in vitro* was determined using pooled hepatic microsomal fractions (final protein concentration of 0.5 mg/mL) at a final test compound concentration of 3 μmol/L.

⑫ Time-resolved fluorescence resonance energy transfer binding affinity assays were performed for BRD4 as previously described.

⑬ The first-in-human trial of drug involves exposure to a single oral dose followed by safety and pharmacokinetic monitoring before subjects progress to an ongoing continuous-dosing phase.

⑭ Computational ocking was performed with AutoDock.

⑮ A mixture solution of three purified proteins was prepared by reconstituting lyophilized protein powder in PBS.

课后练习与讨论

1. 实验方法在写作中有哪些注意要点？
2. 如何评估一篇文章中实验方法部分的写作质量？
3. 如何评估一篇文章的补充材料是否充分恰当？其写作的要点是什么？

第 9 章 ●○

论文格式规范及检查

药学专业论文的投稿材料主要为正文手稿以及相应的补充材料，研究者们都知道，在写作过程中必须遵循一定的专业规范和期刊要求。但是，这些材料的准备通常是由多人在一定时限内完成的，错误或遗漏难以避免，不规范之处时有发生。因此，在投稿前要深刻理解专业论文的格式规范要求，并对这些材料进行细致的检查，确保论文手稿及相应的材料中数据准确、格式规范、语言流畅、图表清晰，达到杂志出版的要求和论文发表的目的。

9.1 药学专业论文的格式规范

药学专业论文的格式规范包括多个方面，以下列举了常见的内容。本节将主要介绍在专业药学英语论文中需要注意的一些语法规则，以及参考文献引用的格式规范。

① 掌握药学论文英文写作的语法规则，避免句型和表达的常见错误。

② 规范引用参考文献及罗列参考文献的格式要求。

③ 熟悉英文标点符号（逗号、句号、分号、冒号、括号、破折号、连字符等）的规范运用，熟练运用大小写、斜体、特殊字体和缩略语等编辑风格。

④ 正确使用数字、数学和度量单位。

⑤ 合理使用图形、图片及表格。

⑥ 遵循药学学科惯例、化学结构编辑，以及化合物编号规则等。

9.1.1 科技论文英文写作的语法规则

（1）主谓一致原则

在一个句子中，主语及其动词在数量上必须保持一致。然而在写作过程中，主谓不一致的错误还是相当普遍，主要原因是主谓语被其他介词间隔开、语序的改变，以及对药学学科主语数量的理解偏差所导致的混淆不清。

① 当一个或多个介词短语出现在主语和动词之间时，或者当句子按照介词短语、动词、主语的顺序构造时，主语的数量可能令人费解，需要

仔细辨别。

例9-1：Successful generation of a T cell-mediated immunity to eliminate antigen includes but it is not limited to the following steps. [主语为 generation]

例9-2：To the intermediate were added THF and NaH. [主语为 THF and NaH]

② 由"and"连接的两个或多个单数主语组成复合主语，相应的谓语动词应为复数形式。然而，形式上为复数但实际上是单数的主语，其对应的谓语动词应为单数形式，这是因为该复合主语已经具备了单一含义。另外，包含"each"和"every"这些词修饰的复合主语采用单数动词。如果复合主语的两个或多个组成部分都没有明确地或含蓄地包含"each"和"every"的意思，则谓语动词必须采用复数形式。

例9-3：The aqueous solubility and hERG inhibition profile of this compound were also viewed as offering a good starting point. [主语为 solubility and profile]

例9-4：Drug discovery and development is a complex, high octane, high risk and potentially highly rewarding endeavor. [复合主语 discovery and development 具备了单一含义]

③ 当两个或多个主语被"or"连接时，动词取决于较近或最近的主语数量，此为"就近原则"。

例9-5：All of the body weights or the mean body weight was recorded.

④ 集合名词（majority、range、couple、number、series、dozen、variety、group）既可以是单数，也可以是复数。当与"the"连用时，表示指代一个整体，该情况下需采用单数动词。当集合中的个体作主语时，集合名词采用复数动词，它们前面往往加"a"修饰。

例9-6：The control group plays an essential role in several clinical studies and serves as standard or baseline for ascertaining the effectiveness of the study drug.

例9-7：A number of key challenges were addressed including off-target kinase selectivity and cardiovascular safety.

⑤ 计量单位被视为集合名词，采取单数动词。

例9-8：Ten miligrams of Pd/C was added to the solution.

⑥ 当分数作为主语的一部分时，谓语动词的单复数取决于主语名词的单复数。

例9-9：Two-third of solvent was evaporated on rotovap.

例9-10：14.1% of Patients were 20～44 years old, 54.0% were 45～64 years old, and 31.8% were≥65 years old.

⑦ "Data" 既可以是单数名词，也可以是复数名词，取决于上下文。

⑧ 以 "ics" 结尾的名词和表示科学学科的名词通常是单数的。

Dynamics   kinetics   thermodynamics   thermokinetics

biophysics   bioinformatics   cheminformatics

（2）避免动词和辅助动词遗漏

复合句中的每一个主语都必须有与之匹配的动词或助动词。

错误：The palladium catalyst was added to the flask, and the mixture stirred at reflux overnight.

正确：The palladium catalyst was added to the flask, and the mixture was stirred at reflux overnight.

（3）限定性表达和非限定制性表达

① 当短语或从句对主句的修饰是必不可少的时候，它就是限定性的；也就是说，没有短语或从句，主语就会变得毫无意义或意义不明。限定性从句最好是用 "that" 而不是 "which" 引出，如果删除以 "that" 开头的从句，主句就不能够传达出有意义的信息。同样地，短语也可以是限定性的。

例9-11：It can be seen that each of the compounds showed pronounced tumor growth inhibition in the two mutant models.

例9-12：Approaches that directly control cellular protein levels have the potential to offer cellular efficacy not easily achievable with small-molecule inhibitors.

例9-13：The PROTAC model for induced protein turnover requires the existence of a ternary complex between the target protein, the PROTAC, and the E3 ligase.

② 如果短语或从句只是增加了主句的信息，但并不是不可或缺的，则是非限定性的；也就是说，如果短语或从句被删除，主句所表达的意义依然完整。非限制性从句可以由"which"或"who"引入，但不能由"that"引入，与主句之间须用逗号隔开。

例9-14：The excitatory neurotransmitter glutamate induces modulatory actions via the metabotropic glutamate receptors (mGlus), which are class C G protein–coupled receptors (GPCRs).

例9-15：We describe the discovery of the clinical candidate AZD9291, a potent EGFR inhibitor.

例9-16：Factor Xa, a trypsin-like serine protease, is crucial to the conversion of prothrombin to thrombin.

（4）悬垂修饰与独立结构

悬垂修饰是指一个修饰词或短语没有与相关联的对象关联起来，以至于它"悬在"空中，是英文写作中常见的语法错误。这是因为在科技论文写作中往往使用被动语态，导致悬垂修饰时有发生。

① 如果一个修饰语在主语之前，它必须修饰那个主语，并用逗号与主语分开。否则，它就是一个悬垂修饰，导致语意不清。

错 误：Using the technology of PROTAC, the targeted protein was efficiently degraded.

正确：Using the technology of PROTAC, we were able to efficiently degrade the targeted protein.

② 在某些情况下，被动语态可以用来纠正悬垂修饰语。

错误：After removing the aqueous layer, the combined organic layers were concentrated.

正确：After the aqueous layer was removed combined, the combined organic layers were concentrated.

③ 以"based on"开头的短语必须修饰紧接在短语前面或后面的名词或代词，而使用以"on the basis of"开头的短语来修饰动词。

错误：Based on cell potency, free fraction, and aqueous solubility, compounds were prioritized.

正确：On the basis of cell potency, free fraction, and aqueous solubility, compounds were prioritized.

独立结构是一种语法结构，涉及一个非限定分句，该分句以附属的形式出现并修饰整个句子，但跟主句没有语法联系，通常以 concerning、considering、given、regarding 等词语开头。独立结构与垂悬结构容易混淆，它们的区别在于，垂悬修饰短语是试图修饰一个特定的名词，却错误地修饰了另一个名词，而独立结构是一个独立的分句，不试图修饰任何名词。如果动作既不是主语发出的，也不是宾语发出的，那么使用独立结构可以避免修饰垂悬。

例9-17：Considering the ability of phthalimides to bind to CRBN, our group and others sought to utilize phthalimides as E3 ligase-recruiting ligands to hijack CRBN in order to degrade target proteins of interest.

例9-18：Structure-based drug design seeks to identify and optimize such interactions between ligands and their host macromolecules, given their three-dimensional structures.

9.1.2 参考文献格式

（1）在正文中引用参考文献

① 在常用的专业论文出版物中，一般通过以下三种方式引用参考文献：

第一种，上标数字，如果引用适用于整个句子或从句，则出现在标点符号之后。

例9-19：Several reviews have summarized the progress in the design of MDM2 inhibitors.[1, 5, 22-30]

第二种，在文本行和标点符号内的圆括号中使用斜体数字。

例9-20：It also complements crystallographic studies of the transmembrane domain structures of class A (*11, 12*), B (*13, 14*), and F (*15*) GPCRs.

第三种，按作者姓名和出版年份在标点符号内的括号内（称为作者-日期格式）。如果作者的名字成为了句子的一部分，则引用文献只需将年份放在括号中。如果在同一个地方有多个引用，请根据第一个作者的姓名按字母顺序列出这些引用，后跟逗号和年份，使用分号来分隔单个引用。如果引用同一作者的多篇文献，不要重复作者名，只需在姓名后列出年份，年份以逗号隔开。如果一个作者在同一年中有多个引用文献，则在年份中添加小写字母以区分它们，例如 2020a、2020b 等。

例9-21：The PD-1 mediated suppression mechanisms appear to be complex, including apoptosis, induction of suppressive cytokines, anergy, exhaustion, and Treg induction (Chen and Han, 2015; Zou and Chen, 2008; Zou et al., 2016).

② 在引用数字参考文献时，从[1]开始，在整个论文中连续编号，包括文本中的参考文献以及表、图和其他非文本组件中的参考文献。如果引用被重复，不要给它一个新的编号，而使用原始的引用编号。

③ 每当给作者命名时，如果一个引用有两个作者，请给出两个名称，并用"and"一词连接；如果一个参考文献有两个以上的作者，可以只列出第一个作者名字，后面跟着"et al."。不要在 et al.之前使用逗号。

Allison and Crews[10]   Crews et al. (*8*)

④ 要在一个数字引文系统中列出某个主要作者和不同合著者的参考，请使用主要作者的姓名，后跟"and co-workers" 或 "and colleagues"。

Crews and co-workers[10-14]   Crews and colleagues (*10, 11*)

⑤ 如果在一个位置引用多篇文献，请按升序列出数字，并用逗号分隔（不带空格作为上标，行上有空格），或者如果这些文献是一个系列，请使用短破折号来指示这些数字的范围。

in the literature (*3-5, 10*)   were summarized[2, 5-7]

（2）在文末列举参考文献

作者应对所有参考文献的准确性和完整性负责，所以应该对照原始文档检查每个引用列表的所有部分。

ⅰ 期刊参考文献必须包括作者姓名、期刊简称、出版年份、卷号（如有）、引文首页（也可以是首末页的完整跨度）。

ⅱ 图书参考必须包括作者或编辑姓名、书名、出版商、出版城市和出版年份。

ⅲ 对于书籍和期刊以外的材料，必须提供足够的信息，以便确定来源和位置。

① 美国化学会（*ACS*）期刊的常见格式如下（注意标点符号、空格、粗体、斜体等规范）：

作者 1；作者 2；作者 3 等等. 文章标题. 期刊简称 年份, 卷数, 页码.

例 9-22：

Ohashi, K.; Maruvka, Y. E.; Michor, F.; Pao, W. Epidermal growth factor receptor tyrosine kinase inhibitor-resistant disease. *J. Clin. Oncol.* **2013**, *31*, 1070-1080.

② 其他期刊列举文献规范

有关不同期刊在列举文献所需采用的正确格式，请参阅该期刊对作者的说明。下面以 *Cell*、*Nature* 和 *Science* 为例。

例如：

Cell 格式：Agarwala, S. S., Glaspy, J., O'Day, S. J., Mitchell, M., Gutheil, J., Whitman, E., Gonzalez, R., Hersh, E., Feun, L., Belt, R., et al. (2002). Results from a randomized phase III study comparing combined treatment with histamine dihydrochloride plus interleukin-2 versus interleukin-2 alone in patients with metastatic melanoma. J. Clin. Oncol. *20*, 125-133.

Nature 格式：Bullock, A. N. et al. Structural basis of inhibitor specificity of the human protooncogene proviral insertion site in moloney murine leukemia virus (PIM-1) kinase. *J. Med. Chem.* **48**, 7604-7614 (2005).

Science 格式：A. Satoh et al., *Bioorg. Med. Chem. Lett.* **19**, 5464-5468 (2009).

9.2 论文手稿及补充材料的检查

论文手稿及补充材料中如果有太多的错误或不规范之处，不但会影响审稿人对该论文的理解，还会使他们产生情绪上的不适。严重时会导致直接拒稿。退一步讲，审稿人会觉得研究者在论文写作上粗心大意，在研究过程中可能也不太严谨，从而怀疑论文本身的数据和结论，以至于在审稿过程中采取更加严苛的标准。所以为了避免功亏一篑，研究者必须在投稿前对论文手稿及相关材料进行细致检查，通常的步骤和内容如下。

9.2.1 论文手稿和补充材料的检查步骤

① 首先，所有作者在电子版上独立修改各种常见错误，比如：数据错误及前后不一致、语言表述不清晰、单词拼写错误、格式不规范等。

② 其次，将论文投稿材料特别是论文手稿打印出来进行细致修改。在纸质版中，对论文内容的视觉外观一目了然，如果有分页的图表或太长的段落也立即可见，并利于前后内容的校对。而且，纸质版更有可能发现与语法、单词顺序和结构有关的错误。

③ 再次，从头到尾阅读论文手稿，可以帮助发现在默读情况下难以发现的错误，尤其是在句子的结构以及是否缺少单词等方面。

④ 最后，请专业的同事或朋友检查你的论文手稿，并提供全方位的修改意见。在许多情况下，他们会提供全新的写作思路，发现被作者忽略的错误等。

9.2.2 论文手稿和补充材料的检查内容

（1）确保论文中所有内容和数据都是准确一致的，避免张冠李戴、前后不一

（2）检查论文手稿的可读性和写作逻辑的清晰性

① 注意上一个句子与下一个句之间的逻辑关系，在某些情况下可使用连接词予以明晰（although, further, yet, rather, thus, in addition 等）。

② 清楚地将自己的工作与他人的工作区分开来，以便审稿人和读者能够快速评估论文中的研究成果及其重要性。

③ 句子长度要合适，一般不超过 30 个单词，也不宜一个句子中套用过多从句。

④ 每个段落的长度要适宜，并注意段落之间的逻辑关系。

⑤ 避免模棱两可或缺乏明确性的语言表述。

（3）确认论文手稿遵循了期刊的写作风格要求

（4）修改任何可能存在的拼写错误

① 利用 word（或其他文本编辑软件）的自动拼写检查器，它能帮助作者发现与单词拼写、主谓动词一致、词序、标点符号、不必要的被动形式等有关的错误。

② 拼写检查器只会标亮自带字典中未包含的单词，但通常不会发现以下示例中的错误。因为它们是词典中的单词，但在语句中不具有作者想要表达的含义。

例9-23：The flask was filed（应为 filled）with water.

例9-24：It was different form（应为 from）what was expected.

其他容易混淆的单词如：choose / chose / choice, filed / field, field / filled, then / than, through / trough, with / whit, funded / founded 等。

③ 忽略拼写检查器中已经正确拼写的专业单词的红色下划线。一个技巧是通过手动的方式，添加到自定义的词典中，从而让这些专业词汇正常显示。

④ 注意区分美式和英式部分单词的拼写方式：

center（美式）/centre（英式）　　　　analyze（美式）/analyse（英式）

color（美式）/colour（英式）　　　　favorite（美式）/favourite（英式）

课后练习与讨论

1. 在专业论文写作中，常见的英语表达错误有哪些？该如何避免？
2. 在日常阅读药学文献的过程中，摘抄文中的精句和短语，并结合自己的科研工作进行模仿改写。
3. 检查论文的格式规范时，应该从哪些方面着手？如何确保投稿材料的检查工作高质量完成？
4. 为什么在撰写药学专业论文时需要引用参考文献？在参考文献方面有哪些格式规范要求？
5. 选取最近阅读的一篇药学专业论文，分别用 *ACS*、*Cell*、*Nature*、*Science* 的格式列举参考文献。

第 10 章 •○

论文投稿及审稿意见回复

10.1 论文投稿及回复

论文投稿流程大致分为论文提交前和论文提交后。

（1）论文提交前

作者需考虑和准备以下事项：
① 选择合适的期刊；
② 根据期刊要求撰写论文；
③ 制作图片摘要（Graphic Abstract）和标题页（Title Page）；
④ 准备补充材料；
⑤ 写一封给编辑的投稿信（Cover Letter）；
⑥ 手稿及其他材料的校对。

（2）论文提交后

在药学专业领域，手稿提交给目标期刊后，一般会进行同行评审（peer review）。首先，期刊编辑会对论文的形式和内容做一个初步的评估，一般考量的因素包括：
① 该论文是否符合本期刊的范围和宗旨；
② 是否严格参照了期刊的作者须知；
③ 是否能引起读者的兴趣；
④ 最近是否刊登过类似的论文；
⑤ 该论文的方法是否完整且严谨。

如果所提交的论文都达到了上述这些要求，期刊编辑才会将该论文提交给同行评审。根据论文的研究内容和方向，选择 3～5 名同行评议专家，从专业角度评价论文的质量，提出意见和判定，主编会按评议的结果决定是否适合在本刊发表。不同期刊的审稿周期长短不一，少则几周，多则半年甚至更长的时间。主编将根据同行评议的结果，对论文做出接收与否的决定。

同行评议的结果一般分以下四种情况，作者应该仔细阅读和理解评审意见，并采取相应的应对措施，以使论文能在合理的时间内得以发表。

① 小修（minor revision）
原因：背景信息、格式、语法、参考文献、谱图等方面有些小瑕疵。非英语母语国家作者投稿有时会被要求语言润色。

应对措施：无原则问题下，诚恳接受并逐条回复审稿意见，尽快把修改稿返回给编辑。一般来说编辑会推荐语言润色机构，若无推荐，可选择公认的润色机构进行润色。润色后可在回复编辑的投稿信中以及在正文致谢部分加以说明。

② 大修（major revision）

原因：补充实验数据、修正实验结论、调整论文结构、加强背景调研、改进言语表述等。

应对措施：对于实验数据的补充，应该尽力而为、量力而行；修正实验结论要有理有据、有礼有节；调整论文结构应仔细斟酌、批判吸收；加强背景调研要查漏补缺，做好归纳总结以及比较；若是需改进语言表述，可以寻求英语较好的同行专家的帮助或英文论文写作机构的加工润色。

③ 拒稿（reject）

原因：创新性达不到期刊要求；实验结果与结论不吻合；逻辑性太差；撰写太糟糕等。

应对措施：如果审稿意见的表述为"no longer needed""not encouraged to submit again"则明确表明了期刊的拒稿态度，这时一定不要死缠烂打，明智的做法是选择其他期刊投稿。但如果审稿的表述为"It is not suitable for publication in its current form, however, if you are willing to revise it according to comments from the reviewers, I would like to reconsider my decision."则表示还可能有希望，可以按照编辑和审稿人的建议进行认真修改，修改稿一定要把他们的最大顾虑打消掉，再重新投稿争取一下。

④ 直接接收（accept as it is）　这种情况相对比较少见，一般是因为主编约稿，或者领域内顶尖学者的论文投稿时才可能发生。

10.2　如何写投稿信（Cover Letter）

所谓"投稿信"就是一封写给编辑的自荐信，在这封信中作者需要告诉编辑三件事情。首先，为什么要投稿？其次，编辑为什么要关注这份手稿？最后，表明该稿件不存在潜在的学术冲突。投稿信虽然不会公开，但对于论文的审理过程至关重要，它不是形式化的文件，不能简单套用，必须认真对待。下例是一封供参考的投稿信。

Dear Editors,

We would like to submit the enclosed manuscript entitled with "Design of Small Molecule Autophagy Modulators: A promising druggable strategy" for publication in *Journal of Medicinal Chemistry*.

For multifactorial diseases such as cancer, neurodegenerative disease and infection the initiation and progression refer to multiple receptors or signaling pathway, and the interventions at one of the targets do not always exhibit desired therapeutic effects. Recently, more and more medicinal chemists have realized this problem and there is an increasing readiness to develop multi-target agents that address multiple targets simultaneously for the purposes of higher therapeutic efficacy and (or) improving safety. However, there are few multi-target drugs in market or clinical trials, despite the best efforts of drug researcher. How to avoid blindness and rationally design multiple ligands is a severe challenge that we face.

Recently researches about designed multiple ligands of diverse multifactorial diseases are emerging. Take JMC as an example, just in 2018, there were more than 60 articles published in this journal describing the research of designed multiple ligands. Some successful cases may provide crucial experience for the development of this field. However, we also notice that few perspectives on this field have been published yet, combination, lead generation, optimization of designed multiple ligands and discuss the critical problems that we face in drug development stage. Subsequently, we analyze the physicochemical properties of 118 clinical multi-target drugs and some designed multiple ligands research cases in recent year, in order to provide successful experience for the development of multi-target drugs and rationally turn the basic research into clinical outcomes. We also discuss the emerging technologies about multifunctional molecules, to exploit enormous potential to secure future therapeutic innovation.

No conflict of interest exits in the submission of this manuscript, and manuscript is approved by all authors for publication. I would like to declare on behalf of my co-authors that the work described is original research that has not been published previously. All the authors listed have approved the submission to your journal.

We deeply appreciate your consideration of our manuscript, and we look forward to receiving comments from the reviewers. If you have any questions, please do not hesitate to contact me.

Yours sincerely,

Prof. XXX
Department of Medicinal Chemistry,
XXX University

在这封 Cover Letter 中，第一段首先表明了投稿来意，第二、三段表述了论文的亮点和价值，第四段是论文的主要内容和框架，最后是投稿声明与致谢。在 Cover Letter 中也可向编辑公正地推荐论文的审稿人或由于利益冲突而避免某个审稿人，采纳与否取决于编辑。在文章修回时要写针对性的、新的 Cover Letter 以说明新的来意以及修改内容。

10.3　同行评议（Peer Review）的作用

同行评议的主要作用有：

① 同行评议的审稿意见出于原创，是非常宝贵的学术资源和极其重要的学术交流方式。

② 审稿意见的针对性极强，可以极大提高相关研究工作的整体水平。

③ 审稿意见对于作者完善研究内容、训练科研思维、拓展知识结构、提高专业水平，具有无可替代的作用。

④ 同行评议是一种较为公正客观的评价体系，利于营造健康的学术氛围。

课后练习与讨论

1. 论文的投稿流程是怎样的？需要准备哪些材料？
2. 收到审稿人意见后，如何回复编辑或审稿人？如果直接拒收，是应该继续修改，还是改投其他期刊？
3. 投稿信（Cover Letter）中应该涵盖哪些内容？
4. 选取一篇药学专业论文进行精读，尝试以作者的身份给编辑写一份"Cover Letter"。
5. 你是否了解同行评议？为什么在药学专业论文的发表过程中，同行评议是一种普遍的做法？你有什么样的改进建议？

推荐阅读论文

药物化学方向：

[1] Bissantz C, Kuhn B, Stahl M. A medicinal chemist's guide to molecular interactions[J]. *J. Med. Chem.*, **2010**, 53(14): 5061-5084.

[2] Finlay M R, Anderton M, Ashton S, et. al. Discovery of a potent and selective EGFR inhibitor (AZD9291) of both sensitizing and T790M resistance mutations that spares the wild type form of the receptor[J]. *J. Med. Chem.*, **2014**, 57(20): 8249-8267.

[3] Ferguson F M, Gray N S. Kinase inhibitors: the road ahead[J]. *Nat. Rev. Drug Discov.*, **2018**, 17(2): 353-377.

[4] Souers A J, Leverson J D, Boghaert E R, et al. ABT-199, a potent and selective BCL-2 inhibitor, achieves antitumor activity while sparing platelets[J]. *Nat. Med.*, **2013**, 19(2): 202-208.

[5] Filippakopoulos P, Qi J, Picaud S, et al. Selective inhibition of BET bromodomains[J]. *Nature*, **2010**, 468(7327): 1067-1073.

[6] Pinto D J, Orwat M J, Koch S, et al. Discovery of 1-(4-methoxyphenyl)-7-oxo-6-(4-(2-oxopiperidin-1-yl)phenyl)-4,5,6,7-tetrahydro-1*H*-pyrazolo[3,4-*c*]pyridine-3-carboxamide (apixaban, BMS-562247), a highly potent, selective, efficacious, and orally bioavailable inhibitor of blood coagulation factor Xa[J]. *J. Med. Chem.*, **2007**, 50(22): 5339-5356.

[7] Sofia M J, Bao D, Chang W, et al. Discovery of a β- d-2'-deoxy-2'- α-fluoro-2'- β-C-methyluridine nucleotide prodrug (PSI-7977) for the treatment of hepatitis C virus[J]. *J. Med. Chem.*, **2010**, 53(19): 7202-7218.

[8] Bondeson D P, Mares A, Smith I E, et al. Catalytic *in vivo* protein knockdown by small-molecule PROTACs[J]. *Nat. Chem. Biol.*, **2015**, 11(8): 611-617.

[9] Lai A C, Crews C M. Induced protein degradation: an emerging drug discovery paradigm[J]. *Nat. Rev. Drug Discov.*, **2017**, 16(2): 101-114.

[10] Ostrem J M, Peters U, Sos M L, et al. K-Ras(G12C) inhibitors allosterically control GTP affinity and effector interactions[J]. *Nature*, **2013**, 503(7477): 548-551.

[11] Meng W, Ellsworth B A, Nirschl A A, et al. Discovery of dapagliflozin: a potent, selective renal sodium-dependent glucose cotransporter 2 (SGLT2) inhibitor for the treatment of type 2 diabetes[J]. *J. Med. Chem.*, **2008**, 51(5): 1145-1149.

[12] Zhao Y J, Aguilar A, Bernard D, et al. Small-molecule inhibitors of the MDM2-p53 protein-protein interaction (MDM2 Inhibitors) in clinical trials for cancer treatment[J]. *J. Med. Chem.*, **2015**, 58(3): 1038-1052.

[13] Link J O, Taylor J G, Xu L, et al. Discovery of ledipasvir (GS-5885): a potent, once-daily oral NS5A inhibitor for the treatment of hepatitis C virus infection[J]. *J. Med. Chem.*, **2014**, 57(5): 2033-2046.

[14] Gilan O, Rioja I, Knezevic K, et al. Selective targeting of BD1 and BD2 of the BET proteins in cancer and immunoinflammation[J]. *Science*, **2020**, 368(6489): 387-394.

[15] McDaniel K F, Wang L, Soltwedel T, et al. Discovery of *N*-(4-(2,4-difluorophenoxy)-3-(6-methyl-7-oxo-6,7-dihydro-1*H*-pyrrolo[2,3-*c*]pyridin-4-yl)phenyl)ethanesulfonamide (ABBV-075/Mivebresib), a potent and orally available bromodomain and extraterminal domain (BET) family bromodomain inhibitor[J]. *J. Med. Chem.*, **2017**, 60(20): 8369-8384.

[16] Li C Y, Yap K, Swedberg J E, et al. Binding loop substitutions in the cyclic peptide SFTI-1 generate potent and selective chymase inhibitors[J]. *J. Med. Chem.*, **2020**, 63(2): 816-826.

[17] Hu J, Lin T, Gao Y, et al. The resveratrol trimer miyabenol C inhibits *β*-secretase activity and *β*-amyloid generation[J]. *PLoS One*, **2015**, 10(1): e0115973.

[18] Kyriukha Y A, Afitska K, Kurochka A S, et al. *α*-Synuclein dimers as potent inhibitors of fibrillization[J]. *J. Med. Chem.*, **2019**, 62: 10342-10351.

[19] Paul A, Viswanathan G K, Mahapatra S, et al. Antagonistic activity of naphthoquinone-based hybrids toward amyloids associated with Alzheimer's disease and type-2 diabetes[J]. *ACS Chem. Neurosci.*, **2019**, 10(8): 3510-3520.

[20] Dai W, Zhang B, Jiang X M, et al. Structure-based design of antiviral drug candidates targeting the SARS-CoV-2 main protease[J]. *Science,* **2020,** 368 (6497): 1331-1335.

[21] He Q L, Minn I, Wang Q, et al. Targeted delivery and sustained antitumor activity of triptolide through glucose conjugation[J]. *Angew. Chem. Int. Ed.,* **2016**, 55 (39): 12035-12039.

[22] Fischer E S, Bohm K, Lydeard J R, et al. Structure of the DDB1-CRBN E3 ubiquitin ligase in complex with thalidomide[J]. *Nature,* **2014,** *512* (7512): 49-53.

[23] Cao Q, Shin W S, Chan H, et al. Inhibiting amyloid-beta cytotoxicity through its interaction with the cell surface receptor LilrB2 by structure-based design[J]. *Nat. Chem.,* **2018,** 10 (12): 1213-1221.

药物分析学方向：

[1] Tayri-Wilk T, Slavin M, Zamel J, et al. Mass spectrometry reveals the chemistry of formaldehyde cross-linking in structured proteins[J]. *Nat. Commun,* **2020**, 11(1): 3128.

[2] Liu J, Cheng R, Van Eps N. et al. Genetically encoded quinone methides enabling rapid, site-specific, and photocontrolled protein modification with amine reagents[J]. *J. Am. Chem. Soc.*, **2020**, 142, 17057-17068.

[3] Feider C L, Krieger A, DeHoog R J, et al. Ambient ionization mass spectrometry: recent developments and applications[J]. *Anal. Chem.*, **2019**, 91(7): 4266-4290.

[4] Lomenick B, Hao R, Jonai N, et al. Target identification using drug affinity responsive target stability (DARTS)[J]. *Proc. Natl. Acad. Sci. U. S. A.*, **2009**, 106(51): 21984-21989.

[5] Shende N, Karale A, Bhagade S, et al. Evaluation of a sensitive GC-MS method to detect polysorbate 80 in vaccine preparation[J]. *J. Pharm. Biomed. Anal.*, **2020**, 183, 113126.

[6] Liu W, Dong H, Zhang L, et al. Development of an efficient biosensor for the *in vivo* monitoring of Cu^+ and pH in the brain: rational design and synthesis of recognition molecules[J]. *Angew. Chem. Int. Ed.*, **2017**, 56(51):

16328-16332.

[7] Bonham A J, Hsieh K, Ferguson B S, et al. Quantification of transcription factor binding in cell extracts using an electrochemical, structure-switching biosensor[J]. *J. Am. Chem. Soc.*, **2012**, 134(7): 3346-3348.

[8] Li J, Peng Z, Wang E. Tackling grand challenges of the 21st century with electroanalytical chemistry[J]. *J. Am. Chem. Soc.*, **2018**, 140(34): 10629-10638.

[9] Song Y J, Zhang Y Q, Bernard P E, et al. Multiplexed volumetric bar-chart chip for point-of-care diagnostics[J]. *Nat. Commun,* **2012**, 3(1): 640-643.

[10] Ashenafi D, Van Hemelrijck E, Chopra S, et al. Liquid chromatographic analysis of oxytocin and its related substances[J]. *J. Pharm. Biomed. Anal.*, **2010**, 51(1): 24-29.

[11] Wang J G, Gao L Q, Lee Y M,et al. Target identification of natural and traditional medicines with quantitative chemical proteomics approaches[J]. *Pharmacol. Ther.*, **2016**, 162: 10-22.

[12] Nováková L, Matysová L, Solich P. Advantages of application of UPLC in pharmaceutical analysis[J]. *Talanta*, **2006**, 68(3): 908-918.

[13] McFedries A, Schwaid A, Saghatelian A. Methods for the elucidation of protein-small molecule interactions[J]. *Cell Chem. Biol.*, **2013**, 20(5): 667-673.

[14] Nilsson A, Goodwin R J, Shariatgorji M, et al. Mass spectrometry imaging in drug development[J]. *Anal. Chem.*, **2015**, 87: 1437-1455.

[15] Liu P, Lu M, Zheng Q, et al. Recent advances of electrochemical mass spectrometry[J]. *Analyst*, **2013**, 138(19): 5519-5539.

[16] Tang Y, Chen X, Wang D, et al. Discover and identify unknown alkylation DNA adducts induced by sulfonates using prediction driven-MRM-profiling strategy[J]. *Talanta*, **2021**, 222: 121500.

[17] Tang Y, Wang Z, Li M,et al. Simultaneous quantitation of 14 DNA alkylation adducts in human liver and kidney cells by UHPLC-MS/MS: application to profiling DNA adducts of genotoxic reagents[J]. *J. Pharm. Biomed. Anal.*, **2019**, 166: 387-397.

[18] Xiao S, Guo J, Yun B H, et al. Biomonitoring DNA adducts of cooked meat carcinogens in human prostate by nano liquid chromatography-high resolution tandem mass spectrometry: identification of 2-amino-1-methyl-6-phenylimidazo[4,5-*b*]pyridine DNA adduct[J]. *Anal. Chem.*, **2016**, 88(24): 12508-12515.

[19] Nicolardi S, Joseph A A, Zhu Q, et al. Analysis of synthetic monodisperse polysaccharides by wide mass range ultrahigh-resolution MALDI mass spectrometry[J]. *Anal. Chem.*, **2021**, 93(10): 4666-4675.

[20] Zhou Y, Xu J, Lu N, et al. Development and application of metal-organic framework@GA based on solid-phase extraction coupling with UPLC-MS/MS for the determination of five NSAIDs in water[J]. *Talanta*, **2021**, 225: 121846.

[21] Chumbley C W, Reyzer M L, Allen J L, et al. Absolute quantitative MALDI imaging mass spectrometry: a case of rifampicin in liver tissues[J]. *Anal. Chem.*, **2016**, 88(4): 2392-2398.

[22] Khadka M, Todor A, Maner-Smith K M, et al. The effect of anticoagulants, temperature, and time on the human plasma metabolome and lipidome from healthy donors as determined by liquid chromatography-mass spectrometry[J]. *Biomolecules*, **2019**, 9(5): 200.

[23] Zhang N, Deng W, Li Y, et al. Formic acid of ppm enhances LC-MS/MS detection of UV irradiation-induced DNA dimeric photoproducts[J]. *Anal. Chem.*, **2020**, 92(1): 1197-1204.

药理学方向：

[1] Sanmamed M F, Chen L. A paradigm shift in cancer immunotherapy: from enhancement to normalization[J]. *Cell*, **2018**, 175(2): 313-326.

[2] Jänne P A, Yang J C, Kim D W, et al. AZD9291 in EGFR inhibitor-resistant non-small-cell lung cancer[J]. *N. Engl. J. Med.*, **2015**, 372(18): 1689-1699.

[3] Granhall C, Donsmark M, Blicher T M, et al. Safety and pharmacokinetics of single and multiple ascending doses of the novel oral human GLP-1 analogue, oral semaglutide, in healthy subjects and subjects with type 2 diabetes[J]. *Clin. Pharmacokinet.*, **2019**, 58, 781-791.

[4] Zanetta C, Nizzardo M, Simone C. et al. Molecular therapeutic strategies for spinal muscular atrophies: current and future clinical trials[J]. *Clin. Ther.*, **2014**, 36(1): 128-140.

[5] Aoyagi A, Condello C, Stöhr J, et al. Aβ and tau prion-like activities decline with longevity in the Alzheimer's disease human brain[J]. *Sci. Transl. Med.*, **2019**, 11(490): eaat8462.

[6] Brown C E, Alizadeh D, Starr R, et al. Regression of glioblastoma after chimeric antigen receptor T-cell therapy[J]. *N. Engl. J. Med.*, **2016**, 375(26): 2561-2569.

[7] Shih Y M, Chang Y J, Cooke M S, et al. Alkylating and oxidative stresses in smoking and non-smoking patients with COPD: implications for lung carcinogenesis[J]. *Free Radic. Biol. Med.*, **2021**, 164: 99-106.

[8] Gobert A P, Boutaud O, Asim M, et al. Dicarbonyl electrophiles mediate inflammation-induced gastrointestinal carcinogenesis[J]. *Gastroenterology*, **2021**, 160(4): 1256-1268.

[9] Takahashi Y, Nishimura T, Higuchi K, et al. Transport of pregabalin via L-type amino acid transporter 1 (SLC7A5) in human brain capillary endothelial cell line[J]. *Pharm. Res.*, **2018**, 35(12): 246.

[10] Li X M, Mu P Q, Wen J K, et al. Carrier-mediated and energy-dependent uptake and efflux of deoxynivalenol in mammalian cells[J]. *Sci. Rep.*, **2017**, 7(1): 5889.

[11] Smahi M, De Pooter N, Hollestelle M J, et al. Monitoring unfractionated heparin therapy: lack of standardization of anti-Xa activity reagents[J]. *J. Thromb. Haemost.*, **2020**, 18(10): 2613-2621.

[12] Sun X, Tang S, Hou B, et al. Overexpression of P-glycoprotein, MRP2, and CYP3A4 impairs intestinal absorption of octreotide in rats with portal hypertension[J]. *BMC Gastroenterol*, **2021**, 21(1): 2.

[13] Rao T, Liu Y T, Zeng X C,et al. The hepatotoxicity of polygonum multiflorum: the emerging role of the immune-mediated liver injury[J]. *Acta. Pharmacol. Sin.*, **2021**, 42(1): 27-35.

[14] Liu L, Fu L, Zhang J W, et al. Three-level hepatotoxicity prediction system based on adverse hepatic effects[J]. *Mol. Pharm.*, **2019**, 16(1): 393-408.

[15] Che T, Majumdar S, Zaidi S A, et al. Structure of the nanobody-stabilized active state of the kappa opioid receptor[J]. *Cell*, **2018**, 172(1-2): 55-67.

[16] Druker B J, Tamura S, Buchdunger E, et al. Effects of a selective inhibitor of the Abl tyrosine kinase on the growth of Bcr-Abl positive cells[J]. *Nat. Med.*, **1996**, 2, 561-566.

[17] Pan C, Li B, Simon M C, Moonlighting functions of metabolic enzymes and metabolites in cancer[J]. *Mol. Cell,* **2021,** 81 (18): 3760-3774.

[18] Shi J, Zhao Y, Wang K, Shi X, et al. Cleavage of GSDMD by inflammatory caspases determines pyroptotic cell death[J]. *Nature,* **2015,** 526 (7575): 660-665.

[19] Hui E, Cheung J, Zhu J, et al. T cell costimulatory receptor CD28 is a primary target for PD-1-mediated inhibition[J]. *Science,* **2017,** 355 (6332): 1428-1433.

[20] Goel S, DeCristo M J, Watt A C, et al. CDK4/6 inhibition triggers anti-tumour immunity[J]. *Nature,* **2017,** 548 (7668): 471-475.

[21] Fang S, Suh J M, Reilly S M, et al. Intestinal FXR agonism promotes adipose tissue browning and reduces obesity and insulin resistance[J]. *Nat. Med.,* **2015,** 21 (2): 159-165.

[22] Yan R, Zhang Y, Li Y, et al. Structural basis for the recognition of SARS-CoV-2 by full-length human ACE2[J]. *Science,* **2020,** 367 (6485): 1444-1448.

[23] Ruiz de Galarreta M, Bresnahan E, Molina-Sanchez P, et al. Beta-catenin activation promotes immune escape and resistance to anti-PD-1 therapy in hepatocellular carcinoma[J]. *Cancer Discov.,* **2019,** 9 (8): 1124-1141.

药剂学方向：

[1] Yue H, Xie K, Ji X, et al. Vascularized neural constructs for ex-vivo reconstitution of blood-brain barrier function[J]. *Biomaterials*, **2020,** 245: 119980.

[2] Shin J Y, Yeo Y H, Jeong J E, et al. Dual-crosslinked methylcellulose hydrogels for 3D bioprinting applications[J]. *Carbohydr. Polym.,* **2020,** 238: 116192.

[3] Ouyang L, Armstrong J P K, Lin Y, et al. Expanding and optimizing 3D bioprinting capabilities using complementary network bioinks[J]. *Sci. Adv.,* **2020,** 6(38): eabc5529.

[4] Liu W J, Zhong Z, Hu N, et al. Coaxial extrusion bioprinting of 3D microfibrous constructs with cell-favorable gelatin methacryloyl microenvironments[J]. *Biofabrication,* **2018,** 10(2): 024102.

[5] Tega Y, Tabata H, Kurosawa T, et al. Structural requirements for uptake of diphenhydramine analogs into hCMEC/D3 cells via the proton-coupled organic cation antiporter[J]. *J. Pharm. Sci.,* **2021,** 110: 397-403.

[6] Dąbrowska-Bouta B, Sulkowski G, Frontczak-Baniewicz M, et al. Ultrastructural and biochemical features of cerebral microvessels of adult rat subjected to a low dose of silver nanoparticles[J]. *Toxicology,* **2018,** 408: 31-38.

[7] Hayeshi R, Hilgendorf C. Artursson P, et al. Comparison of drug transporter gene expression and functionality in Caco-2 cells from 10 different laboratories[J]. *Eur. J. Pharm. Sci.,* **2008,** 35(5): 383-396.

[8] Yang H, Sun L, Pang Y, et al. Three-dimensional bioprinted hepatorganoids prolong survival of mice with liver failure[J]. *Gut,* **2021,** 70(3): 567-574.

[9] Kang D, Hong G, An S, et al. Bioprinting of multiscaled hepatic lobules within a highly vascularized construct[J]. *Small,* **2020,** 16(13): e1905505.

[10] Nieskens T T, Wilmer M J. Kidney-on-a-chip technology for renal proximal tubule tissue reconstruction[J]. *Eur. J. Pharmacol.,* **2016,** 790: 46-56.

[11] Li Y, Wu M, Zhang N, et al. Mechanisms of enhanced antiglioma efficacy of polysorbate 80-modified

paclitaxel-loaded PLGA nanoparticles by focused ultrasound[J]. *J. Cell Mol. Med.*, **2018**, 22(9): 4171-4182.

[12] Tan J J Y, Nguyen D V, Common J E, et al. Investigating PEGDA and GelMA microgel models for sustained 3D heterotypic dermal papilla and keratinocyte Co-Cultures[J]. *Int. J. Mol. Sci.*, **2021**, 22(4): 2143.

[13] Xiao C J, Qi X R, Aini W, et al. Preparation of cisplatin multivesicular liposomes and release of cisplatin from the liposomes in vitro[J]. *Acta Pharm. Sin.*, **2003**, 38(2): 133-137.

[14] Abramson A, Caffarel-Salvador E, Khang M, et al. An ingestible self-orienting system for oral delivery of macromolecules[J]. *Science*, **2019**, 363 (6427), 611-615.

[15] Chiang C S, Lin Y J, Lee R, et al. Combination of fucoidan-based magnetic nanoparticles and immunomodulators enhances tumour-localized immunotherapy[J]. *Nat. Nanotechnol.*, **2018**, 13 (8), 746-754.

[16] Ebeid K, Meng X, Thiel K W, et al. Synthetically lethal nanoparticles for treatment of endometrial cancer[J]. *Nat. Nanotechnol.*, **2018**, 13 (1), 72-81.

[17] Farah S, Doloff J C, Muller P, et al. Long-term implant fibrosis prevention in rodents and non-human primates using crystallized drug formulations[J]. *Nat. Mater.*, **2019**, 18 (8), 892-904.

[18] Haque S, Feeney O, Meeusen E, et al. Local inflammation alters the lung disposition of a drug loaded pegylated liposome after pulmonary dosing to rats[J]. *J. Control. Release*, **2019**, 307, 32-43.

[19] Hu C M, Zhang L, Aryal S, et al. Erythrocyte membrane-camouflaged polymeric nanoparticles as a biomimetic delivery platform[J]. *Proc. Natl. Acad. Sci. USA*, **2011**, 108 (27), 10980-10985.

[20] Kim H J, Zhang K, Moore L, et al. Diamond nanogel-embedded contact lenses mediate lysozyme-dependent therapeutic release[J]. *ACS Nano*, **2014**, 8 (3), 2998-3005.

[21] Shahbazi R, Sghia-Hughes G, Reid J L. Targeted homology-directed repair in blood stem and progenitor cells with CRISPR nanoformulations[J]. *Nat. Mater.*, **2019**, 18 (10), 1124-1132.

[22] Yan X, Zhou Q, Vincent M. Multifunctional biohybrid magnetite microrobots for imaging-guided therapy[J]. *Sci. Robot.*, **2017**, 2 (12), eaaq1155.

[23] Yu J, Wang J, Zhang Y, et al. Glucose-responsive insulin patch for the regulation of blood glucose in mice and minipigs[J]. *Nat. Biomed. Eng.*, **2020**, 4(5), 499-506.

推荐阅读书目

[1] Wallwork A. English for Writing Research Papers[M]. Italy: Springer New York Dordrecht Heidelberg London, 2011.

[2] Coghil A M, Garson L R.The ACS Style Guide[M]. New York:Oxford University Press, 2006.

附：药学专业词汇表

A

absorption n. 吸收

absorptivity n. 吸收系数

accumulate v. 累积；积聚

accuracy n. 准确度

acetal n. 乙缩醛

acetonitrile n. 乙腈

acetyl n. 乙酰基

acetylcholine n. 乙酰胆碱

acetylcholinesterase n. 乙酰胆碱酯酶

acid n. 酸

acid-dye colorimetry 酸性染料比色法

acidity n. 酸度；酸性

acquire v. 获得

acquired immune deficiency syndrome 获得
    性免疫缺陷综合征

acquisition n. 获得物；收购

acridine n. 吖啶

activate v. 使活化；激活

activation n. 激活；活化作用

activator n. 活化剂；激活剂

active targeting preparation 主动靶向制剂

activity n. 活动；活性

acute adj. 剧烈的；急性的

acyclic adj. 非环状的；非周期的

acyclovir n. 阿昔洛韦

adaptive adj. 适应性的

addiction n. 成瘾性

addition n. 增加；添加物

additional adj. 附加的；额外的

additive n. 添加剂；添加物

adenosine n. 腺苷

adherence n. 黏附；粘连；依从性

adhesion n. 黏附（力）

adhesive strength 黏附力

adipose n. 脂肪

adjacent adj. 与……毗邻的；邻近的

adjustment n. 调整；调节；调节器

administer v. 管理；施用(药物等)

administration n. 给药；管理；行政机构

adoption n. 采用

adoptive adj. 收养的；采用的

adrenal adj. 肾上腺的

adrenaline n. 肾上腺素

adrenocortical hormone 肾上腺皮质激素

advantage n. 优势；优点

adverse adj. 不利的；相反的

adverse drug reaction 不良反应

affinity n. 亲和力；吸引力；密切关系；
    类同

affinity chromatography 亲和色谱法

agent n. 试剂

agglomeration n. 凝聚；结块

aggregation n. 聚集体；集合体

agonism n. 激动；激动作用

agonist n. 激动剂

alanine n. 丙氨酸

albendazole n. 阿苯达唑

albumin n. 白蛋白；清蛋白

alcohol n. 乙醇；酒精

aldehyde n. 醛

aldol n. 羟醛；羟醛缩合

alendronate   n. 阿仑膦酸钠

aliphatic   adj. 脂肪族的

alkaline   adj. 碱性的

alkalinity   n. 碱度

alkene   n. 烯烃

alkyl   n. 烷基

alkylation   n. 烷基化

alkyne   n. 炔烃

alleviate   v. 减轻；缓和

allosteric   adj. 变构的；别构的

allyl   n. 烯丙基

alprostadil   n. 前列地尔

alternative   n.替换物；
adj.可供选择的

aluminum   n. 铝

alveoli   n. 肺泡

Alzheimer's disease   阿尔茨海默病

amantadine   n. 金刚烷胺

ambient   adj. 周围的

ambroxol   n. 氨溴索

amide   n. 酰胺

amidine   n. 脒

amikacin   n. 阿米卡星

amination   n. 氨基化；胺化

amine   n. 胺

amino   n. 氨基

aminoglycoside   n. 氨基糖苷类

aminophylline   n. 氨茶碱

aminotransferase   n. 氨基转移酶

ammonia   n. 氨；氨水

ammonium   n. 铵

amorphous   adj. 无定形的；无组织的；非
晶形的

amorphous form   无定形

amoxicillin   n. 阿莫西林

amphipathic   adj. 两亲性的

amphotericin B   n. 两性霉素 B

amplification   n. 放大；扩大

amplify   v. 放大；扩大

amylin   n. 胰岛淀粉素

analgesics   n. 镇痛药

analogue   n. 类似物

analysis   n. 分析；验定

analyte   n. 待测物

analytical quality control（AQC）   分析质
量控制

anatomy   n. 解剖；解剖学

anchor   v. 锚定

androgen   n. 雄激素

anemia   n. 贫血

angio-   adj. 血管的

angiogenesis   n. 血管生成

angiotension converting enzyme inhibitor
（ACEI）   血管紧张素转化酶抑制药

angstrom   n. 埃（光谱线波长单位）

anhydride   n. 酸酐

anhydrous   adj. 无水的

aniline   n. 苯胺

anion   n.阴离子

anionic   adj. 阴离子的；带负电荷离子的

antacid   n. 抗酸药

antagonism   n. 拮抗作用

antagonist   n. 拮抗剂

antiangiogenic   adj. 抗血管生成的

antiasthmatic drug   平喘药

antibacterial activity   抗菌活性

antibacterial spectrum   抗菌谱

antibiotic   adj. 抗菌的；
n. 抗生素

antibiotic drugs   抗菌药

antibiotic   n. 抗生素

antibody   n. 抗体

antiemetic　n. 止吐药

antifibrinolysin　n. 抗纤维蛋白溶酶

antifungal agents　抗真菌剂

antigen　n. 抗原

antioxidant　n. 抗氧化剂

anti-proliferative　adj. 抗细胞增生的

antitussive　n. 止咳药

antiviral　adj. 抗病毒的

apoptosis　n. 细胞凋亡

apparatus　n. 仪器；装置

applicable　adj. 可适用的；可应用的

approach　n. 方法；

　　　　　　v. 靠近；接近

approval　n. 批准；认可

approximately　adv. 大概；大约

aqueous　adj. 水的；含水的

area normalization method　面积归一化法

arginine　n. 精氨酸

argon　n. 氩气

aromatic　adj. 芳香的；芳香族的

aromatic water　芳香水剂

arrhythmia　n. 心律失常

artemisinin　n. 青蒿素

artery　n. 动脉

arthr/o　adj. 关节的

artificial　adj. 人造的；仿造的

aryl　n. 芳烃基

arylation　n. 芳基化

aseptic technique　无菌操作法

asparaginase　n. 天冬酰胺酶

asparagine　n. 天冬酰胺

aspirin　n. 阿司匹林

assay　n. 试验；含量测定

assessment　n. 评价；评估

assumption　n. 假定；假设

asymmetric　adj. 不对称的

asymmetrical stretching vibration　不对称伸缩振动

atherosclerosis　n. 动脉粥样硬化

atmospheric pressure ionization　大气压离子化

atom　n. 原子

atomic absorption spectrophotometry　原子吸收分光光谱法

atomic emission spectrophotometry　原子发射光谱法

atropine　n. 阿托品

attenuate　v.减弱；稀薄

　　　　　adj. 减弱的；稀薄的；细小的

audio-　adj. 听觉的

augment　n. /v. 增加；增大

autacoid　n. 自体活性物质

autoimmune　adj. 自身免疫的

autosampler　n. 自动进样器

auxiliary　adj. 辅助的；备用的

auxochrome　n. 助色团

available　adj. 可获得的；有空的

azeotrope　n. 恒沸物；共沸混合物

azetidine　n. 氮杂环丁烷；吖丁啶

azole　n. 唑类

B

Bacillus Calmette-Guerin　卡介苗

backbone　n. 骨架

bacterial drug resistance　细菌耐药性

bactericidal drug　杀菌药

bacteriostatic drug　抑菌药

bacterium　n. 细菌（bacteria pl.）

band width　谱带峰宽

bar graph　棒图

base　n. 基础；碱

baseline　n. 基线

basic　adj. 基础的；碱的

basicity　n. 碱度；碱性

beam   n. 光束

beclomethasone   n. 倍氯米松

bend   v. /n. 弯折

benproperine   n. 苯丙哌林

benzene   n. 苯

benzimidazole   n. 苯并咪唑

benzisoxazole   n. 苯异噁唑

benzodiazepine   n. 苯二氮䓬类

benzofuran   n. 苯并呋喃

benzopyran   n. 苯并吡喃

benzoquinone   n. 苯醌

benzothiophene   n. 苯并噻吩

benzotriazole   n. 苯并三氮唑

benzoxazole   n. 苯并噁唑

benzoyl   n. 苯甲酰基

benzyl   n. 苯甲基；苄基

benzylpenicillin   n. 苄青霉素

between-run precision   批间精密度

bicyclic   adj. 二环的

bilayer   n. 双分子层

bind   v. 结合，捆绑

bioactive   adj. 生物活性的

bioavailability   n. 生物利用度

biocompatibility   n. 生物相容性；生物适
   合性

biodegradation   n. 生物降解

bioequivalence test   生物等效性试验

bioinformatics   n. 生物信息学

bioisostere   n. 生物电子等排体

biology   n. 生物；生物学

biomarker   n. 生物标志物

biomaterial   n. 生物材料

biomedical   adj. 生物医学的

biopharmaceutical analysis   体内药物分析

biopsy   n. 活组织检查；穿刺活检

biotin   n. 生物素；维生素H

bisphosphonate   n. 磷酸盐

bleach   v. （使）漂白；（使）褪色

block   v. 阻止；阻塞；阻断

blood-brain barrier   血脑屏障

bloodstream   n. 体内循环的血液

boiling range   沸程

bond   n. 键；联结

   v. 成键；连接

bonding   n.键合；黏合

bone marrow   骨髓

boronate   n. 硼酸酯

borylation   n. 硼化

boundary   n. 边界；界限

branched   adj. 分支的；分部的；血管分
   支的

brine   n. 卤水；盐水

   v. 用浓盐水处理

bromhexine   n. 溴己新

bromide   n. 溴化物

bronchia   n. 支气管

baseline correction   基线校正

buffer   n. [计] 缓冲区；缓冲器

   v. 缓冲

buffer capacity   缓冲容量

buffer solution   缓冲溶液

bulk   n. 体积；容量；大部分

bulk density   堆密度

bulky   adj. 体积大的

buret   n. 滴定管

butyl   n. 丁基

bypass   n. 旁路；支路

   v.绕过；绕开

byproduct   n. 副产物

C

cardiac   adj. 心脏的

calcineurin inhibitor 钙调神经磷酸酶抑制剂

calcitonin   n. 降钙素

calcitriol   n. 钙三醇

calcium   n. 钙（Ca）

calibration   n. 校正

calibration curve   校正曲线

camptothecin   n. 喜树碱

computer-aided drug design（CADD）   计算机辅助药物设计

cancer   n. 癌症

capacity   n. 能力；容量；资格；地位；生产力

capillary   n. 毛细管

carbamate   n. 氨基甲酸酯

carbazochrome   n. 卡巴克洛

carbazole   n. 咔唑

carbocation   n. 碳正离子

carbohydrate   n. 碳水化合物；糖类

carbon   n. 碳

carbonate   n. 碳酸盐

carboxylate   n. 羧酸盐

carboxylic acid   羧酸

carcino-   n. 癌

carcinogen   n. 致癌物质

carcinoma   n.肿瘤；癌

cardiac glycoside   n. 强心苷

cardiovascular   adj. 心血管的

carrier   n. 载体

cascade   n. 级联

caspofungin   n. 卡泊芬净

catecholamine   n. 儿茶酚胺

catalysis   n. 催化作用；催化

catalyze   v. 催化

cation   v. 阳离子

cation exchange resin 阳离子交换树脂

cationic   adj. 阳离子的
　　　　　　n.阳离子

cefazolin   n. 头孢唑林

celite   n. 硅藻土

cell   n. 细胞

cell cycle   细胞周期

cell line   n. 细胞系

cellular   adj. 细胞的；多孔的；由细胞组成的

central nervous system（CNS）   中枢神经系统

centrifugation   n. 离心法

centrifuge   n. 离心机
　　　v. 用离心机分离；使……受离心作用

cephalosporin   n. 头孢菌素

cephradine   n. 头孢拉定

cerebral   adj. 大脑的

ceriometry   n. 铈量法

cesium   n. 铯（Cs）

channel   n. 途径；频道；通道

chaperone   n. 分子伴侣

characteristic frequency   特征频率

characterization   n. 描述；特性描述

characterized   adj. 以……为特点的

charge   n. 费用；电荷
　　　　　　v. 使充电

checkpoint   n. 检查点；关卡

chelate   n. 螯合物

chemical approach   化学方法

chemical shift   化学位移

cheminformatics   n. 化学信息学

chemokine   n. 趋化因子

chemotherapeutic index   化疗指数

chemotherapy   n. 化学疗法

chiniofon   n. 喹碘方

chiral   adj. 手性的

chiral separation   手性分离

chiral stationary phase   手性固定相

chirality   n. 手性

chloramphenicol　n. 氯霉素

chloride　n. 氯化物

chlorine　n. 氯（Cl）

chloroform　n. 三氯甲烷；氯仿

chloroquine　n. 氯喹

chlortetracycline　n. 金霉素

choleic　adj. 胆的

cholesterol　n. 胆固醇

choline　n. 胆碱

chopper　n. 切光器

chromatin　n. 染色质

chromatogram　n. 色谱图

chromatography　n. 色层分析；色谱分析法

chromophore　n. 发色团

chromosome　n. 染色体

chronic　adj. 慢性的；长期的

cimetidine　n. 西咪替丁

ciprofloxacin　n. 环丙沙星

circumference　n. 圆周；周长

cirrhosis　n. 硬化；肝硬化

cisplatin　n. 顺铂

clarity　n. 澄清度

clearance　n. 清除率

cleavage　n. 分裂；解理

clinical pharmaceutics　临床药剂学

clinicopathological　adj. 临床病理的

clone　n. 克隆；无性繁殖

　　　　　v. 无性繁殖

clopidogrel　n. 氯吡格雷

coagulant　n. 促凝血药

coagulation　n. 凝固；凝结

cochlear　adj. 耳蜗的

codeine　n. 可待因

coefficient of variation　变异系数

collagen　n. 胶原，胶原质

collapse　n. 崩溃；倒塌；病倒；

v.（肺或血管）萎陷；（尤指因病重而）倒
　　下；昏倒

colloid　n. 胶体
　　　　　adj. 胶状的

colloidal　adj. 胶体的；胶态的

colon　n. 结肠

colorimetric　adj. 比色的；色度的

colorimetry　n. 比色法

column overload　柱超载

combination　n. 组合；结合；化合

compartment　n.区室；分室

compatibility　n. 兼容性

compatible　adj. 能兼容的；可共处的

competitive　adj. 竞争性的

complex　adj. 复杂的；合成的

complexometric titration　络合滴定

component　n. 组成部分；成分；元件
　　　　　adj. 组成的；构成的

composition　n. 成分；组成

compound　n. 化合物；混合物；复合词
　　　　　v. 合成；混合；恶化；加重

compound medicine　复方药

compression　n. 压缩，浓缩；压迫

concentration　n. 浓度；浓缩

concerted　adj. 协同的；协调的

concomitant　n. 伴随物
　　　　　adj. 相伴的；共存的

condensation　n. 浓缩

condenser　n. 冷凝管

conductivity　n. 导电性

confidence interval　置信区间

confidence level　置信水平

configuration　n. 构型

confirm　v. 确认；确定；证实

confocal　adj. 共焦的；同焦点的

conformation　n. 构象

conjugate n. /v. 共轭

conjugation n. 共轭

constant n. 常数；恒量

constant weight 恒重

constitution n. 构造

content n. 含量；内容

controllability n. 可控性

controlled adj. 可控的；克制的

coordination number 配位数

copolymerization n. 共聚作用

copper n. 铜

core n. 核心；要点

cornea n. 角膜

coronary heart disease n. 冠心病

correlation coefficient 相关系数

corticotrophin n. 促肾上腺皮质激素

cortisol n. 皮质醇

cortisone n. 可的松

coumarin n. 香豆素

counterfeit medicine 假药

coupling n. 偶联

covalent adj. 共价的

cranial adj. 颅的

cretinism n. 克汀病

cross-coupling 偶联

crucible n. 坩埚

crude n. 粗品；石油

crude drug 生药

crystal n. 晶体

　　　　adj. 晶体的

crystal form 晶型

crystal structure 晶体结构

crystallization n. 结晶

crystallize v. 结晶

culture n. 文化；栽培

　　　　v.（细胞）培养

cumulative adj. 累积的

cumulative size distribution 累积分布

curable adj. 可治愈的；可医治的

curvature n. 曲率；弯曲

curvette cell 比色池

cyano adj. 含有氰基的

cyclic voltammetry 循环伏安法

cycloalkyl n. 环烷基

cyclohexane n. 环己烷

cyclooxygenase n. 环氧酶

cyclopentane n. 环戊烷

cyclophosphamide n. 环磷酰胺

cyclopropyl n. 环丙基

cyclosporin n. 环孢菌素

cyclooxygenase n. 环氧化酶

cysteine n. 半胱氨酸

cystic adj. 膀胱的

cytochrome P450 细胞色素 P450

cytokine n. 细胞因子

cytomembrane n. 细胞膜

cytometry n. 血细胞计数

cytoplasm n. 细胞质

cytoplasmic adj. 细胞质的

cytoskeletal adj.细胞支架的

cytoskeleton n. 细胞骨架；细胞支架

cytosol n. 细胞溶质

cytotoxic adj. 细胞毒素的

cytotoxicity n. 细胞毒性

D

dactinomycin n. 放线菌素

dapsone n. 氨苯砜

data n. 数据；资料

database n. 数据库

day to day precision 日间精密度

de novo 从头合成

decarboxylation 脱羧

decomposition n. 分解；变质

decrease　v. 减少；减小；降低

　　　　　n. 减少；减小；减少量

deficiency　n. 缺乏；缺失

definition　n. 定义

degasser　n. 脱气器

degenerative　adj. 恶化的；退化的

degradable　adj. 可能降解的

degrade　v. 降解；退化；使降解

degree　n. 程度；度

dehydrase　n. 脱水酶

dehydrocholic acid　去氢胆酸

deionized water　去离子水

deletion　n. 删除；遗失

deliver　v. 交付；发表；递送；释放；实

　现；传送；履行；投递

delivery　n. 递送；分娩

demonstrate　v. 证明；展示；论证

demonstration　n. 示范；证明

denaturation　n. 变性

densitometry　n. 光密度法

density　n. 密度

dentistry　n. 牙科

deoxygenation　n. 脱氧

deplete　v. 耗尽；用尽；使衰竭

deprotection　n. 去保护

derivative　n. 衍生物；派生物

derive　v. 源于；得自；获得

dermato-　adj. 皮肤的

dermis　n. 皮肤；真皮

desiccant　n. 干燥剂

desiccate　v. 干燥

desiccator　n. 干燥器

deuterium　n. 氘

develop　v. 开发；发展

deviation　n. 偏差

device　n. 装置

dextran　n. 右旋糖酐

dextrin　n. 糊精；葡聚糖

dextromethorphan　n. 右美沙芬

dextrose　n. 右旋糖；葡萄糖

diabetes　n. 糖尿病

diabetes mellitus　糖尿病

diagnose　v. 诊断；判断

diagnostic　adj. 诊断的

　　　　　　n. 诊断法

dialysis　n. 透析；渗析

dialyze　v. 透析

diameter　n. 直径

diastereomer　n. 非对映异构体

diazapam　n. 地西泮

dicoumarol　n. 双香豆素

dielectric constant　介电常数

diene　n. 二烯

dienophile　n. 亲二烯体

differential scanning calorimetry （DSC）
　差示扫描量热法

differential spectrophotometry　差示分光光
　度法

differential thermal analysis（DTA）　差示
　热分析法

differentiation　n. 分化

diffusion　n. 传播；扩散

digestion　n. 消化；领悟

diguanidine　n. 双胍类

dihedral　n. 二面角

　　　　　adj. 有两个平面的

dilute　v. 稀释

　　　　adj. 稀释的

dimer　n. 二聚体

diode　n. 二极管

dioxane　n. 二噁烷

dipolar　adj. 两极的

discharge　v. 放电；排出

disintegrant　n. 崩解剂

disk assemble method　圆盘法

disorder　n. 紊乱

　　　　　v. 使失调

dispense　v. 发给，配药

dispersal　n. 分散；传播；散布

disperse　v. 分散；传播

　　　　　adj. 分散的

disperse medium　分散介质

disperse phase　分散相

disperse system　分散体系

dispersed　adj. 分散的；散布的

dispersing device　色散装置

display　n. /v. 显示

disposition　n. 处置

dissociation　n. 分离；解离

dissolution　n. 分解；溶解

dissolve　v. 溶解

distal　n. 末梢的；末端的

distillation　n. 蒸馏

distilled water　蒸馏水

distribution　n. 分配；分布

disulfide　n. 二硫化物

diuretic　n. 利尿药

docking　n. 对接

domain　n. 结构域

donepezil　n. 多奈哌齐

dosage　n. 剂量

dose　n. 剂量

　　　　v. 给药

dose-dependent　剂量依赖的

double-blind test　双盲测试

doxorubicin　n. 多柔比星

doxycycline　n. 多西环素

drop　n. 滴；微量；滴剂

　　　　v. 滴落；下降；终止

dropper　n. 滴管

dropwise　adv. 逐滴地；一滴一滴地

drug carrier　药物载体

drug design　药物设计

drug quality control　药品质量控制

druggability　n. 成药性

drug-like　类药；类药性

dry oven　干燥箱

drying to constant weight　干燥至恒重

duplicate　v.复制；重复

durability　n. 耐用度；持久

dye　n. 染料；染色

　　　　v. 把……染上颜色；被染色

dynamics　n. 力学

E

effect　n. 效果；影响；作用　v. 影响

effective　adj. 有效的；起作用的

effectively　adv. 有效地

effector　n. 效应器

efficacy　n. 效能

efficacy　n. 功效；效能

ejection　n. 喷出

elastic deformation　弹性变形

elastic recovery（ER）　弹性复原率

elastic work　弹性功

elasticity　n. 弹性

electrochemisty　n. 电化学

electrode　n. 电极

electromagnetic radiation　电磁辐射

electron　n. 电子

electron-deficient　缺电的

electron-donating　供电子

electronegativity　n. 电负性

electronic balance　电子天平

electron-rich　富电子的

electron-withdrawing　吸电子的

electrophile　n. 亲电试剂

electrophoresis　n. 电泳

electrospray ionization　电喷雾电离

electrostatic　adj. 静电的

element　n. 元素；要素；原理；成分

elemental　adj. 基本的；主要的

　　　　　　n. 基本原理

eliminate　v. 消除；排除

elimination　n. 消除；排泄

ellipsoid　n. 椭圆体

elongation　n. 延长；伸长

eluant　n. 洗脱剂；淋洗剂

elusive　adj. 难懂的；难捉摸的

elute　v. 洗脱

embolization　n. 栓塞（现象）

emission　n.（光、热等的）发射

emulsification　n. 乳化；乳化作用

enamine　n. 烯胺

enantiomer　n. 对映体

enantioselective　adj. 对映选择性的

enantioselectivity　n. 对映选择性

encapsulate　v. 封装；形成胶囊

encephalic　adj. 脑的

encode　v. 编码

endocytosis　n. 内吞

endogenous　adj. 内生的；内源性的

endogenous substances　内源性物质

endothelial　adj. 内皮的

endothelin　n. 内皮素

endpoint　n. 终点

engulfment　n.吞噬；吞入

enhance　v. 提高；加强；增加

enol　n. 烯醇

enolization　n. 烯醇化

ensure　v. 确定；保证

enteral　adj. 肠的

enthalpy　n. 焓

entity　n. 实体；本质

entrapment　n. 包埋；截留

entropy　n. 熵

enzyme　n. 酶

enzyme immunoassay　酶免疫分析

ephedrine　n. 麻黄碱

epidemic　adj. 传染性的；流行性的

epidermal growth factor receptor（EGFR）
　表皮生长因子受体

epigenetic　adj. 表观遗传的；后生的

epilepsy　n. 癫痫

epimer　n. 差向异构体

epithelial　adj. 上皮的

epoxidation　n. 环氧化

epoxide　n. 环氧化物

equation　n. 方程式；相等；反应式

equilibrium　n. 平衡

equilibrium constant　平衡常数

equimolar　n. 等摩尔

equivalent　n. 当量

　　　　　　adj. 等量的

ergot　n. 麦角

error and variation　误差和变异

erythrocytic stage　红细胞内期

erythrocyte　n.红细胞；红血细胞

erythropoietin　n. 促红细胞生成素

escape　v. 逃避；避开

　　　　　n. 逃跑；泄漏

esophagus　n. 食管

ester　n. 酯

estrogen　n. 雌激素

ethanol　n. 乙醇

ether　n. 醚

ethical（prescription）drug　处方药

ethinylestradiol　n. 炔雌醇

ethyl　n. 乙基

evaporate　v. 蒸发

evaporation　n. 蒸发

evolution　n. 演变；进化

ex vivo　体外；离体

excipient　n. 辅料

excitation　n. 激发

excitation spectrum　激发光谱

exclusion chromatography　排阻色谱

excrete　v. 排泄；分泌

exhaustion　n. 枯竭；耗尽；精疲力竭

exoerythrocytic stage　红细胞外期

expansion　n. 膨胀；阐述；扩张物

expectorant　n. 祛痰药

experimental　adj. 实验的

expose　v. 揭露；使曝光；显示

extend　v. 延伸；扩大

external phase　分散介质；外相；连续相

extracellular　adj. 细胞外的

extracted ion chromatogram　提取离子流图

extraction　n. 萃取

extrude　v. 挤出；压出

F

fabrication　n. 构造

facilitate　v. 促进；帮助；使容易

factor　n. 因子；因素

far IR　远红外

fast atom bombardment　快原子轰击

fasting　n. 禁食；斋戒
　　　　adj. 空腹的

feature　n./v. 特征

feces　n. 粪便

feedback　n. 反馈

female　adj. 雌性的
　　　　n. 雌性动物

fermentation　n. 发酵

ferric ammonium citrate　枸橼酸铁铵

ferrous sulfate　硫酸亚铁

fibrinolytic drugs　纤维蛋白溶解药

fibroblast　n. 纤维原细胞；成纤维细胞

fibrosis　n. 纤维化

field desorption ionization　场解吸离子化

field ionization　场电离

filament　n. 单纤维

filariasis　n. 丝虫病

film　n. 薄膜；电影
　　　v. 在……上覆薄膜

filter　n. 过滤器

filtrate　n. 滤液

filtration　n. 过滤

flask　n. 烧瓶

flavone　n. 黄酮

flavonoid　n. 类黄酮

flow curve　流动曲线

flow velocity　流出速度

fluconazole　n. 氟康唑

flucytosine　n. 氟胞嘧啶

fluorescence　n. 荧光

fluorescence efficiency　荧光效率

fluorescence life time　荧光寿命

fluorescence quantum yield　荧光量子产率

fluoride　n. 氟化物

fluorine　n. 氟

fluorometer　n. 荧光计

fluorometry　n. 荧光分析法

fluorophore　n. 荧光基团

fluorouracil　n. 氟尿嘧啶

flutamide　n. 氟他胺

folic acid　n. 叶酸

food and drug administration（FDA）　美国
　　食品药品管理局

formation n. 形成；构造；编队

formula n. 公式；分子式

formulation n. 制剂，配方

fourier transform ion cyclotron resonance mass spectrometry 傅里叶变换离子回旋共振质谱仪

fraction collector 馏分收集器

fragment n. 碎片

frameshift adj. 基因移码的

frequency n. 频率；频繁

fructose n. 果糖

function n. 函数；功能

functional adj. 功能的

functional group 官能团

functionalization n.功能化；官能团化

functionalize v. 使功能化；使起作用；给化合物增加功能团

fungus n. 真菌

funnel n. 漏斗

furan n. 呋喃

furosemide n. 呋塞米

fusion n. 融合；融合物

fusion method 热熔法

G

gametocyte n. 配子体；配子母细胞

ganglion n. 神经节

gas chromatography （GC）气相色谱

gas chromatography-mass spectrometry （GC-MS） 气相色谱-质谱联用

gaseous ion 气态离子

gastric adj. 胃部的

gastric ulcer 胃溃疡

gastrointestinal adj. 胃肠的

gatifloxacin n. 加替沙星

gel n. 凝胶
      v. 胶化

general identification test 一般鉴别试验

generate v. 使形成；发生；生殖

genome n. 基因组

genotoxicity n. 基因毒性

genotype n. 基因型；遗传型

gentamicin n. 庆大霉素

glomerulus n. 肾小球

glucagon n. 胰高血糖素

glucocorticoid n. 糖皮质激素

glucose n. 葡萄糖

glutamine n. 谷氨酰胺

glutathione n. 谷胱甘肽

glycine n. 甘氨酸

glycol n. 乙二醇

glycomics n. 糖组学

glycoprotein n. 糖蛋白

good clinical practice（GCP） 药物临床试验质量管理规范

good laboratory practice（GLP） 药品实验室管理规范

good manufacturing practice（GMP） 药品生产质量管理规范

good supply practice（GSP） 药品供应管理规范

G-protein coupled receptor（GPCR） G 蛋白偶联受体

gradient n. 梯度

gram n. 克

granule n. 颗粒

granule density 颗粒密度

granulocyte n. 粒细胞；粒性白细胞

gravimetric method 重量法

growth fraction 生长比率

guanidine n. 胍

gutzeit 古蔡氏法

gynaecological adj. 妇科的；妇科学的

H

hemagglutinin　n. 血凝素

haemoglobin　n. 血红蛋白；血色素

half peak width　半峰宽

half-time　n. 半衰期

halide　n. 卤化物

halogen　n. 卤素

head space concentrating injector　顶空浓缩
进样器

healthcare product　保健产品

heart failure　n. 心力衰竭

heavy metal　重金属

helix　n. 螺旋；螺旋状物

hematological　adj. 血液学的

hemi-homolysis cleavage　半均裂

hemoglobin　n. 血红蛋白；血红素

heparin　n. 肝素

hepatic　adj. 肝的

hepatitis　n. 肝炎

hepatocellular　adj. 肝细胞的

hepatocyte　n. 肝细胞

hereditary　adj. 遗传的

heterocycle　n. 杂环

heterogeneity　n. 异质性；不均匀性

heterogeneous　adj. 多相的；不均一的

heterolytic cleavage　异裂（非均裂）

high performance liquid chromatography-
mass spectrometry（HPLC-MS）高效
液相色谱-质谱联用

high-throughput screening（HTS）高通量
筛选

histamine　n. 组胺

histamine receptor antagonist　组胺受体拮
抗剂

histidine　n. 组氨酸

histocompatibility　n. 组织相容性

histological　adj. 组织学的

histology　n. 组织学

histone　n. 组蛋白

holographic grating　全息光栅

homeostasis　n. 稳态

homogeneous　adj. 单一的；均匀的

homogenize　v. 使均匀；搅匀

homolytic cleavage　均裂

hormone　n. 激素；荷尔蒙

hormone replacement therapy　激素替代疗法

human immunodeficiency virus（HIV）人
类免疫缺陷病毒

humidity　n. 湿度；湿气

hybrid　n. 杂化；混合
adj. 混合的

hybridization　n. 杂化；杂交

hybridization affect　杂化影响

hydrogen　n. 氢

hydrogen bond　氢键

hydrogen-ion activity　氢离子活度

hydrogenolysis　n. 氢解作用

hydrolyze　v. 水解

hydrolysis　n. 水解作用

hydrophile-lipophile balance（HLB）亲
水-亲油平衡值

hydrophilicity　n. 亲水性

hydrophobic　adj. 疏水的

hydrophobicity　n. 疏水性

hydrotropy agent　助溶剂

hydroxyl　n. 羟基

5-hydroxytryptamine　n. 5-羟色胺

hypercholesterolaemia　高胆固醇血症

hyperchromic effect　增色效应

hyperglycemia　n. 高血糖症

hypertension　n. 高血压

hypochromic effect　减色效应

hypotonic   adj. 低渗的

hypoxia   n. 低氧

I

IC$_{50}$ 半数抑制浓度

identification   n. 鉴别

identification test   药物鉴别试验

illumination   n. 照明

image   n. 影像

imatinib   n. 伊马替尼

imidazole   n. 咪唑

imidazoline   n. 咪唑啉

imine   n. 亚胺

immersion   n. 浸润；陷入

immobile liquid   不可流动液体

immune   adj. 免疫的

immunity   n. 免疫

immunohistochemistry   免疫组织化学

immunology   免疫学

immuno-oncology   免疫肿瘤学

immunostimulant   n. 免疫刺激剂

immunosuppressant   n. 免疫抑制剂

impurity   n. 杂质；不纯

in vitro   离体；体外

in vivo   在体；体内

incident plane   入射平面

inclusion compound   包含物

incubate   v. 孵化；培养

indazole   n. 吲唑

indicator   n. 指示剂

indole   n. 吲哚

infect   v. 感染；传染

infectious   adj. 传染的

infiltrate   n. 渗透物
            v. 渗入

inflammation   n. 炎症

inflammatory   adj. 发炎的；炎症的

infrared spectrophotometry   红外分光光度法

infrared spectroscopy   红外吸收光谱法

infusion   n. 灌输；浸泡；注入物

ingredient   n. 原料；要素；组成部分

inhalation   n. 吸入剂；吸入

inherent   adj. 固有的；内在的；与生俱来的

inhibitor   n. 抑制剂

initial   adj. 最初的
          n. 原始细胞

injection   n. 注射

injection port   进样口；气化室

inoculation   n. 接种

in-plane bending vibration   面内弯曲振动

insomnia   n. 失眠

instability   n. 不稳定（性）

instillation   n. 滴剂；滴注

insulin   n. 胰岛素

intact   adj. 完整的

integrate   v. 使……完整；使……成整体
            adj. 整合的；完全的

intensity   n. 强度

interface polycondensation   界面缩聚法

interference   n. 干扰；冲突；干涉

interferon   n. 干扰素

interleukin   n. 白介素

intermediate   n. 中间体

internal   adj. 内部的

internal conversion   内转换

internal standard method   内标法

internalization   n. 细胞内化

interval   n. 间隔

intestine   n. 肠

intracellular   adj. 细胞内的

intraperitoneal   adj. 腹腔的

intravenous   adj. 静脉的

intrinsic activity   n. 内在活性

iodide   n. 碘化物

iodine   n. 碘（I）

ion   n. 离子

ion abundance   离子丰度

ion source   离子源

ion trap   离子阱

ion-exchange resin   离子交换树脂

ionization   n. 离子化

ipriflavone   n. 依普黄酮

iron   n. 铁

irreversible   adj. 不可逆的

isobutyl   n. 异丁基

isocratic elution   等度洗脱

isoelectric focusing   等电点聚焦

isoflavone   n. 异黄酮

isoleucine   n. 异亮氨酸

isomer   n. 同分异构体

isoniazid   n. 异烟肼

isoprenaline   n. 异丙肾上腺素

isopropyl   n. 异丙基

isoquinoline   n. 异喹啉

isotope   n. 同位素

isotopic ion   同位素离子

isoxazole   n. 异噁唑

K

kanamycin   n. 卡那霉素

ketoconazole   n. 酮康唑

ketone   n. 酮

kidney   n. 肾脏

kinase   n. 激酶

kinetic   adj. 动能的

kinetics   n. 动力学

kinin   n. 激肽

knock down   基因敲低

knock in   基因敲入

knock out   基因敲除

L

label   v. 标记；示踪

labeled amount   标示量

lactam   n. 内酰胺

lactate   n. 乳酸；乳酸盐

lactone   n. 内酯

Lag time   滞留时间

lamivudine   n. 拉米夫定

laxative   n. 泻药

layer   n. 层；膜

lead   n. 先导化合物；铅

lethal   adj. 致死的

leucine   n. 亮氨酸

leukemia   n. 白血病

leukotriene   n. 白三烯

level   n. 水平；标准
          adj. 水平的；平坦的
          v. 瞄准；拉平；使同等

levofloxacin   n. 左氧氟沙星

levorotatory   adj. 左旋的

ligand   n. 配位体；配基

ligase   n. 连接酶

light source   光源

light-scattering   光散射

lignan   n. 木酚素

limit of detection   检测限

limit of quantitation   定量限

linearity and range   线性与范围

lingual   adj. 舌的

lipophilic   adj. 亲酯的

lipophilicity   n. 亲脂性

lipoxygenase   n. 脂氧酶

liquid chromatography（LC）   液相色谱

liquid paraffin 液体石蜡

liquid-solid extraction 液固提取法

lithium n. 锂（Li）

litmus paper 石蕊试纸

liver n. 肝脏

long-term testing 长期试验

lubricate v. 润滑

lymphocyte n. 淋巴细胞

lysine n. 赖氨酸

M

macromolecule n. 大分子

macrophage n. 巨噬细胞

magnesium n. 镁（Mg）

magnesium sulfate n. 硫酸镁

magnetic-sector mass spectrometer 磁质谱仪

malaria n. 疟疾

male adj. 雄性的

　　　 n. 雄性

malignant adj. 恶性的

malignant neoplasm 恶性肿瘤

manganese n. 锰（Mn）

mass spectrum 质谱图

mass-to-charge ratio 质荷比

matrix-assisted laser desorption ionization
　基质辅助激光解吸电离

maximum n. 最大值

mebendazole n. 甲苯咪唑

mechanism n. 机理；机制

medical device 医疗器械

medication n. 药物；药物治疗

medium n. 培养基

melanoma n. 黑色素瘤

melt v. 熔化；融解

membrane n. 膜；薄膜

meninges n. 脑脊膜

mercury n. 汞

mesylate n. 甲磺酸盐

meta adj. 转移；间位；在后

metabolic adj. 新陈代谢的

metabolism n. 新陈代谢

metabolite n. 代谢物

metastable peak 亚稳峰

metastasis n. 转移

metformine n. 二甲双胍

methanol n. 甲醇

methionine n. 甲硫氨酸；蛋氨酸

methodology n. 方法学；方法论

methotrexate n. 甲氨蝶呤

methoxyl n. 甲氧基

methyl n. 甲基

methyl red 甲基红

methylation n. 甲基化

methylene n. 亚甲基

methyltestosterone n. 甲睾酮

metronidazole n. 甲硝唑

microburet n. 微量滴定管

micrometre n. 微米

micromolar adj. 微摩尔的

microscopy n. 显微镜检查

microsomal n. 微粒体

microwave spectrum 微波谱

milligram n. 毫克

mineralocorticoid n. 盐皮质激素

minimum n. 最小值

minimum detectable concentration 最低检
　出浓度

minimum detectable quantity 最低检出量

mitochondrial adj. 线粒体的

mitomycin n. 丝裂霉素

mitotic adj. 有丝分裂的

mobile phase 流动相

modification   n. 修饰；改变

modify   v. 修饰；改变

moiety   n. 一部分

moisture   n. 水分；潮湿

molar   adj. 摩尔的

molar absorptivity   摩尔吸收系数

molecular weight   分子量

molecule   n. 分子

molybdenum   n. 钼（Mo）

monoclonal   adj. 单克隆的

monocyte   n. 单核细胞

monotherapy   n. 单一疗法

morphine   n. 吗啡

morpholine   n. 吗啉

morphology   n. 形态学

mortality   n. 死亡率；死亡数

motif   n. 基序

moxifloxacin   n. 莫西沙星

multidrug resistence   n. 多药耐药性

multiple   adj. 多重的；许多的

　　　　　　n. 倍数；并联

multi-targeted   adj. 多靶点的

murine   n. 鼠科动物

　　　　　adj. 鼠的

muscarine   n. 毒蕈碱

mutant   adj. 突变的

mutation   n. 突变

myel-   adj. 脊髓的

my（o）-   adj. 肌肉的

myxedema   n. 黏液性水肿

N

nalidixic acid   萘啶酸

nasal   adj. 鼻的

national formulary   国家处方集

neoplastic   adj. 瘤的

neostigmine   n. 新斯的明

nephr（o）-   adj. 肾的

neural   adj. 神经的

neuraminic acid   n. 神经氨酸

neurodegeneration   n. 神经退行性变

neuropathy   n. 神经病

neurotransmitter   n. 神经递质

nicotine   n. 烟碱

nithiocyanamine   n. 硝硫氰胺

nitration   n. 硝化

nitric oxide   一氧化氮

nitrile   n. 腈

nitrofurantoin   n. 呋喃妥因

nitrogen   n. 氮

nitroglycerin   n. 硝酸甘油

non-nucleotide reverse transcriptase inhibitor
　　　非核苷逆转录酶抑制剂

nonpolar   adj. 非极性的

non-steroidal anti-inflammatory drug   非甾
　　　体抗炎药

norfloxacin   n. 诺氟沙星

normal phase   正相

normalization   归一化法

nuclear   adj. 细胞核的

nuclear magnetic resonance spectroscopy
　　　（NMR）   核磁共振

nucleophile   n. 亲核试剂

nucleophilic   adj. 亲核的

nucleoside   n. 核苷

nucleus   n. 细胞核

O

obesity   n. 肥胖

ocular   adj. 眼的

ofloxacin   n. 氧氟沙星

oligomer   n. 低聚体

omeprazole　n. 奥美拉唑

oncogene　n. 癌基因

oncogenic　adj. 致癌的

oncology　n. 肿瘤学

oocyst　n. 卵囊

optical isomer　光学异构体

optimization　n. 优化

optimize　v. 优化

oral　adj. 口腔

organ　n. 器官；机构

organic volatile impurities　有机挥发性杂质

ortho　n. 邻位

orthogonal test　正交试验

oscillate　v. 振荡；振动

oseltamivir　n. 奥司他韦

osteo　adj. 骨的

osteonectin　n. 骨粘连蛋白

over the counter（OTC）　非处方药

overexpression　n. 过表达

oxalate　n. 草酸；草酸根

oxaliplatin　n. 奥沙利铂

oxazole　n. 噁唑

oxetane　n. 氧杂环丁烷

oxidation　n. 氧化作用

oxidation-reduction titration　氧化还原滴定

oxime　n. 肟

oxygen　n. 氧（O）

oxytocin　n. 缩宫素；催产素

P

P-glycoprotein　n. P-糖蛋白

palladium　n. 钯（Pd）

pancreas　n. 胰腺

pancreatin　n. 胰酶

pancreatitis　n. 胰腺炎

para-　n. 对位

paradigm　n. 范例；词形变化表

parameter　n. 参数

parasympathetic nerve　副交感神经

parathyroid hormone　甲状旁腺激素

Parkinson's disease　帕金森病

partial least squares method（PLS）　偏最
小二乘法

partition coefficient　分配系数

parts per million　百万分之

pathogen　n. 病原体

pathology　n. 病理学

patient　n. 病人；患者
　　　　　adj. 有耐心的

peak area　峰面积

peak height　峰高

pellet　n.小丸；丸剂

penetrate　v. 穿透；渗入

penicillin　n. 青霉素

pepsin　n. 胃蛋白酶

peptic ulcer　消化性溃疡

peptide　n. 肽

permeability　n. 渗透率；渗透性

phagocytosis　n. 吞噬作用

pharmaceutical analysis　药物分析

pharmaceutics　n. 药剂学

pharmacodynamics　n. 药效学

pharmacokinetics　n. 药物代谢动力学

pharmacology　n. 药理学

pharmacophore　n. 药效团

pharmacopoeia　n. 药典

pharmacy　n. 药学

phenol　n. 苯酚

phenolphthalein　n. 酚酞

phenomenon　n. 现象

phenotype　n. 表现型

phentolamine　n. 酚妥拉明

phenyl　n. 苯基

phenylalanine　n. 苯丙氨酸

phosphate　n. 磷酸盐

phospholipase　n. 磷脂酶

phosphorus　n. 磷

phosphorylation　n. 磷酸化

photodiode array detector　光二极管阵列检

　测器

photon　n. 光子

photostability　n. 耐光性

physicochemical　adj. 物理化学的

physiochemical property　理化性质

physiology　n. 生理学

pilocarpine　n. 毛果芸香碱

pinacol　n. 频哪醇

pipemidic acid　吡哌酸

piperazine　n. 哌嗪

piperidine　n. 哌啶

pipet　n. 吸量管；移液管

pitocin　n. 催产素

pituitary　n. 垂体

pituitrin　n. 垂体后叶激素

placebo　n. 安慰剂

plasma　n. 血浆

plasmodium　n. 疟原虫

platelet　n. 血小板

pneumonia　n. 肺炎

polar　adj. 极性的

polarity　n. 极性

polymerase　n. 聚合酶

polymorphism　n. 多形态

polypeptide　n. 多肽

polysaccharide　n. 多糖

post antibiotic effect　抗生素后效应

potassium　n. 钾（K）

potency　n. 效价；效力

potential　n. 潜能；势能；电位；电势

potentiometric titration　电位滴定

powder　n. 粉；粉末

　　　　 v. 撒粉；使成粉末

praziquantel　n. 吡喹酮

precipitate　v. 沉淀

　　　　　 n. 沉淀物

precipitation　n. 沉淀

precision　n. 精密度

preclinical　adj. 临床前的

preparation　n. 准备；制备

preserve　v. 保存

pretreatment　n. 预处理

prism　n. 棱镜

prodrug　n. 前药

progestogen　n. 孕激素

proliferation　n. 增殖；增生

proline　n. 脯氨酸

proof-of-concept　概念验证阶段

property　n. 性质；性能

propranolol　n. 普萘洛尔

prostaglandin　n. 前列腺素

prostate　n. 前列腺

protease　n. 蛋白酶

protease inhibitor　蛋白酶抑制剂

protecting group　保护基团

protein　n. 蛋白

protein tyrosine kinase　蛋白质酪氨酸激酶

proteolysis　n. 蛋白质水解

protonation　n. 质子化作用

psychiatric disorder　精神失常

psycho-　adj. 心理的

pulmonary　adj. 肺的

pupil　n. 瞳孔

purification　n. 纯化

purine　n. 嘌呤

purity   n. 纯度；纯净

pyran   n. 吡喃

pyrazine   n. 吡嗪

pyrazole   n. 吡唑

pyridazine   n. 哒嗪

pyridine   n. 吡啶

pyridone   n. 吡啶酮

pyrimethamine   n. 乙胺嘧啶

pyrimidine   n. 嘧啶

pyrogen   n. 致热源

pyrrole   n. 吡咯

pyrrolidine   n. 吡咯烷

quality   n. 质量；特性

quality evaluation   质量评价

quality standard   质量标准

quantification   n. 定量；量化

quantity   n. 量；数量

quench   v. 淬灭；熄灭；猝灭

quinestrol   n. 炔雌醚

quinine   n. 奎宁

quinoline   n. 喹啉

quinolone   n. 喹诺酮

R

racemate   n. 外消旋体

racemic   adj. 外消旋的

racemization   n. 外消旋作用

radical   n. 自由基
         adj. 激进的；根本的

radiotherapy   n. 放射疗法

raloxifene   n. 雷洛昔芬

raman scattering light   拉曼光

ranitidine   n. 雷尼替丁

react   v. 反应

reaction   n. 反应

reactivity   n. 反应性

reagent   n. 试剂

rearrangement   n. 重排

receptor   n. 受体

recombinant   adj. 重组的

recovery   n. 回收率

recrystallization   n. 重结晶

rectum   n. 直肠

red shift   红移

reduction   n. 减少；还原

reductive   adj. 具还原性的

reference electrode   参比电极

reference substance   标准（对照）物质

reflux   v. 回流

refractive index   折光系数

regiospecific   adj. 区域专一性的

relative humidity（RH）   相对湿度

renal   adj. 肾脏的

renewability   n. 可再生性

repeatability   n. 重复性

replication   n. 复制；回答

replicon   n. 复制子

representative   adj. 典型的；有代表性的
               n. 代表；典型

reproducibility   n. 重现性

resolution   n. 分辨率；解决；决心

resonance   n. 共振

respiration   n. 呼吸

retention   n. 保留；滞留

retina   n. 视网膜

reverse transcriptase   逆转录酶

reverse-phase   反相

reversible   adj. 可逆的；可反转的

reyleigh scattering light   瑞利光

rhodamine   n. 罗丹明（红色荧光染料）

ribavirin   n. 利巴韦林

rifampin   n. 利福平

rigidity　n. 硬度；刚性

rinse　v. 漱；冲洗掉；漂净

rocking vibration　面内摇摆振动

rodent　n. 啮齿动物

rotamer　n. 旋转异构体

rotovap　旋转蒸发仪

roxithromycin　n. 罗红霉素

S

salbutamol　n. 舒喘灵；沙丁胺醇

sample　n. 样品；样本

sample injection valve　进样阀

structure-activity relationship（SAR）　构
效关系

scaffold　n. 骨架

scattering light　散射光

scavenger　n. 食腐动物；清道夫；
清除剂；拾荒者

schematic　n. 原理图

scheme　n. 方案；计划

sedimentation　n. 沉积（作用）

selective estrogen receptor modulators　选择
性雌激素受体调节剂

sensitivity　n. 敏感；灵敏度

sequential　adj. 连续的；有顺序的

serine　n. 丝氨酸

serotonin　n. 血清素

serum　n. 血清

side chain　侧链

side effect　n. 副作用

signal to nosie（S/N）　信噪比

significant figure　有效数字

sildenafil　n. 西地那非

silica gel　硅胶

silver　n. 银

sirolimus　n. 西罗莫司

sodium　n. 钠

sodium bicarbonate　碳酸氢钠

solubility　n. 溶解度；溶解性

soluble　adj. 可溶解的

solution　n. 溶液

solvent　n. 溶剂

specific identification test　专属鉴别试验

specific rotation　比旋度

specificity　n. 特异性；专一性

spectral line　谱线

spectrograph　n. 光谱仪

spectrophotometry　n. 分光光度法

spectroscopy　n. 光谱学

spectrum　n. 光谱

spiro　n. 螺环

stability　n. 稳定性

stabilize　v. 使稳定

standard deviation（SD）　标准差

standard operating procedure（SOP）　标准
操作流程

state-of-the-art　adj. 当今技术水平的

statin　n. 他汀类

statistics　n. 统计

steatohepatitis　n. 脂肪性肝炎

stereochemistry　n. 立体化学

stereoisomer　n. 立体异构体

stereoselectivity　n. 立体选择性

stereospecific　adj. 立体专一性的

stereospecificity　n. 立体专一性

sterilize　v. 杀菌；消毒

steroid　n. 类固醇

stir　v. 搅拌

stir bar　搅拌棒

stock solution　储备液

stoichiometric　adj 化学计量的

stoichiometric point　化学计量点

stomach n. 胃

strain n. 张力；菌株

v. 拉紧

streptomycin n. 链霉素

stretching vibration 伸缩振动

strong band 强带

structure n. 结构

substituent n. 取代基

adj. 被替代的

substrate n. 底物

subtype n. 亚型

sucralfate n. 硫糖铝

sulfate n. 硫酸盐

sulfonamide n. 磺胺类药

sulfone n. 砜

sulfonyl n. 磺酰基

sulfoxide n. 亚砜

sulfur n. 硫

sulfonylurea n. 磺酰脲类

sumatriptan n. 舒马普坦

supercritical fluid chromatography（SFC）
超临界流体色谱法

superposition n. 叠加；重叠

suppress v. 抑制；镇压

susceptibility n. 易感性

suspension n. 悬浮；混悬液

symmetric adj. 对称的

symmetrical stretching vibration 对称伸缩
振动

symmetry n. 对称性

sympathy n. 交感神经

symptom n. 症状；征兆

syndrome n. 综合症状；并发症状

synergistic adj. 协同的

synthesis n. 合成；综合

synthetic adj. 合成的

system suitability 系统适用性

T

tailing n. 拖尾

tailing peak 拖尾峰

tamoxifen n. 他莫昔芬

tandem mass spectrometry 串联质谱

target n. 靶点

tautomer n. 互变异构体

temperature n. 温度；体温

tensile strength（Ts） 抗张强度

teriparatide n. 特立帕肽

terpenoid n. 萜类化合物

test solution 试液

testosterone n. 睾酮

tetracycline n. 四环素

tetrahydrofuran n. 四氢呋喃

tetrazole n. 四氮唑

thalamus n. 丘脑

therapeutic drug monitoring 治疗药物监测

thermodynamics n. 热力学

thermogravimetric analysis 热重分析

thermometer n. 温度计

thiazide n. 噻嗪类

thiazole n. 噻唑

thickness n. 厚度；层；浓度

thin layer chromatography（TLC） 薄层色
谱法

thiol n. 硫醇

thiophene n. 噻吩

thiouracil n. 硫脲嘧啶

threonine n. 苏氨酸

thrombin n. 凝血酶

thrombocytopenia n. 血小板减少（症）

thromboxan n. 血栓素

thyroglobulin n. 甲状腺球蛋白

thyroid gland   n. 甲状腺

thyroxine   n. 甲状腺素

ticagrelor   n. 替格瑞洛

ticlopidine   n. 噻氯匹定

time-of-flight mass spectrometry   飞行时间
质谱仪

tinidazole   n. 替硝唑

tissue   n. 组织

titrant   n. 滴定剂

titration curve   滴定曲线

titrimetry   n. 滴定法

tobramycin   n. 妥布霉素

tolerance   n. 耐受性

toluene   n. 甲苯

topochemical reactions   局部化学反应

torsion   n. 扭转

tosylate   n. 甲苯磺酸盐

total ion current chromatogram   总离子流图

toxicity   n. 毒性

toxicology   n. 毒物学；毒理学

trace amount   痕量

trachea   n. 气管

traditional Chinese medicine   中药

transcription   n. 转录

transdermal   adj. 经皮的；经皮肤

transduction   n. 转导

transition   n. 过渡；转换

translocation   n. 易位

transmembrane   adj. 跨膜的

transmembrane transport   跨膜转运

transmitted light   透射光

transplant   v. 移植

transporter   n. 转运体

trial   n. 试验；审讯

triazole   n. 三唑类

trifluoromethyl   n. 三氟甲基

trigger   v. 触发；引起

triglyceride   n. 甘油三酯

triiodothyronine   n. 三碘甲状腺氨酸

tritium   n. 氚

tryptophan   n. 色氨酸

tuberculosis   n. 结核病

tumor   n. 肿瘤

turbidimetric assay   浊度测定法

turbidimetry   n. 比浊法

turbidity   n. 浑浊度；浑浊性

twisting vibration   蜷曲振动

tyrosine   n. 酪氨酸

tyrosine hydroxylase   酪氨酸羟化酶

U

ubiquitin   n. 泛素

ultracentrifugation   n. 超速离心

ultraviolet-visible spectrophotometry   紫外-
可见分光光度法

uniformity of dosage unit   含量均匀度

uptake   v. 吸收；摄取

urea   n. 尿素

ureter   n. 输尿管

urethra   n. 尿道

ursodeoxycholic acid   熊去氧胆酸

V

vaccine   n. 疫苗

vacuum   n. 真空

validate   v. 证实；验证

valine   n. 缬氨酸

vapor pressure   蒸气压

vascular   adj. 血管的；脉管的

venule   n. 小静脉

versatility   n. 多功能性

vertebral   adj. 椎骨的

vessel   n. 血管；容器

viability   n. 活性；生存能力

vibrational relexation   振动弛豫

vinblastin   n. 长春花碱

vinyl   n. 乙烯基

virus   n. 病毒

viscosity curve   黏度曲线

visual comparison   目视比色法

vitamin   n. 维生素

void ratio   空隙比

volumetric flask   容量瓶

W

warfarin   n. 华法林

wave number   波数

wavelength   n. 波长

whole blood   全血

X

xenograft   n. 异种移植

Y

yeast   n. 酵母

yield   n. 产量；产率
         v. 产出

Z

zalcitabine   n. 扎西他滨

zidovudine   n. 齐多夫定

zwitterion   n. 两性离子